CANDIDA CURE:

HEALING NATURALLY IN 90 DAYS

Over 5,000 Successful Cases!

Dr. George J. Georgiou, Ph.D.,D.Sc (AM).,N.D.

Published by:
Da Vinci Health Publishing
Panayia Aimatousa 300
Aradippou 7101
Larnaca
Cyprus

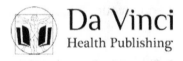

Da Vinci
Health Publishing

MEDICAL DISCLAIMER: The following information is intended for general information purposes only. Individuals should always see their health care provider before administering any suggestions made in this book. Any application of the material set forth in the following pages is at the reader's discretion and is his or her sole responsibility.

ISBN - 978-9925-569-02-1

Dedication:

First, I would like to bow deeply to the thousands of patients who have helped me understand the complexities of Candida and who need to take credit for the time spent with them in refining this protocol over many years.

All these patients over the years have been my "laboratory" for developing many treatment protocols through trial and error, backed by research.

I would also like to thank all the researcher scientists, lecturers and teachers who dedicate their life to helping others, and all the courageous health professionals who go against the grain of the establishment, while thinking outside the box.

A loving hug of gratitude to my wife and 4 children for their support and understanding during my professional endeavours throughout these years – they are all blessed.

Finally, I deeply embrace the Divine faith that I have been blessed with, that has helped me believe in the innate healing abilities of the body, through the power of Natural healing, without chemical intervention.

A profound blessing to you all and may your healing journey be fruitful and fulfilling!

TABLE OF CONTENTS

CHAPTER 1:

Curing My Own Candida

Before we begin discussing the details of the Candida protocol that I invented some years ago, let me take you on a health odyssey of what motivated me to spend many hundreds of hours investigating Candida and its related problems.

Despite all my knowledge in biology and the workings of the human body after completing an initial degree in the Biological Sciences in the UK, by the time I had reached the age of 30 my health was a shamble.

I could just about manage to crawl out of bed with excruciating pain in my body and band-type headaches that would last most of the day. I would have a painful breakfast with many digestive issues, drag myself to my office, see patients for a couple of hours, then go back to bed for 2-3 hours before seeing a few more patients in the afternoon. Painkillers and anti-inflammatories were my main support to get through the day.

At the time, I was working as a Clinical Psychologist and Clinical Sexologist; apart from the biology degree, I also had qualified in these too. I had not discovered the wonderful world of natural medicine at this time, but this was all going to change in the next few years.

By evening time, I was too tired to do anything, and it required a concerted effort just to hold a conversation. I tended to avoid company for this reason and became a recluse – living life close to my devoted family and trying to enjoy the small moments of watching my children develop. I absolutely hated the way I was. By nature, I am a "Type A" personality who loves to be on the go, researching new things – I generally have a very inquisitive mind and like people.

After many months of these persistent symptoms, including chronic headaches that would last for days, accompanied by an unexplainable fatigue, I eventually went to the local G.P. who took some X-rays and found that my frontal sinuses were loaded with fluid – he immediately prescribed antibiotics. Less than two months later I was back there again for more antibiotics as my sinuses were again blocked and causing headaches and pain, not to mention the tiredness, apathy, and on occasions depression. I was quite incapacitated, and this was certainly enough to cause an active person to fall into a depression – I used to love my work. There is nothing more frustrating than waking every morning with band-type headaches that prevented me from concentrating on my work.

Erratic Performance and Behavior

It was around the same time that I was also invited to teach part-time at a local flight school – they wanted me to teach the psychological factors around safety and communication to budding pilots who were passing exams for their Private Pilot's License (PPL).

These topics combine both psychology and biology, so I was duly suited, having degrees in both. I had no qualms about accepting this job offer as one of my deepest passions while still at school was to

2

become an RAF jet pilot. But as fate would have it, there were other plans for me. It was not long before the school invited me to take my own PPL. They felt that this would facilitate my teaching, as it would give me the experience of being in the cockpit. I was ecstatic!

I needed no further persuading – I began ground school immediately and within a short while I was sitting in the left-hand seat flying a Cessna 152 and a Piper Cherokee. But the problem that my instructors could never understand was why my flying was so erratic.

On my "good" days when I would get up feeling generally clear-headed and alert, I would fly the plane to perfection with perfect take-offs and landings as we practiced our touch-and-goes. On the "bad" days when I would get up with a headache, sore muscles, lack of sleep and generally feeling like a truck had run over me, I would sit in the cockpit ready for take-off and upon applying full power, I could hardly steer straight on the runway – much to my instructor's horror! There were many days that he was having kittens! Eventually I got my license, but it was a tough uphill climb (literally!), with the instructor's blood pressure seeing better times.

To cut a long story short, in the 7 years of frequenting various medics, allergy specialists and an ENT surgeon (who eventually persuaded me to have a septum operation for a supposedly defective septum in my nose), I was in a much worse state than when I first began getting symptoms. In these 7 years, I had taken 18 courses of antibiotics and was in a real mess.

My symptoms had now worsened and became more frequent, including headaches and migraines, fibromyalgia (pains and aches in all my body), chronic fatigue (or Myalgic Encephalitis as it was diagnosed by one homeopathic doctor), bowel distension, more or less constant stomach pains with dreadful distension, Leaky Gut Syndrome, Systemic Candidiasis with skin itching, rashes, chronic tiredness and more.

3

I sought diagnosis and treatment abroad in the US and the UK. I was getting weaker and weaker and was now becoming ill with whatever, I ate. I was getting desperate as my workload and obligations grew – I now had a family with two young children and was building a house, as well as conducting many additional professional duties. Despite ill health, I was invited to do a radio programme and I accepted; I was also asked to write a column in a national tabloid with a large circulation, and I accepted that too. I could barely manage to keep going, but my wife stood beside me and helped whenever possible.

Seeking Help from Natural Medicine

In desperation, I began reading Natural Medicine books. I was fumbling in the dark as even though my initial degrees were in biology and psychology, I had not really delved into the fascinating science of Natural Medicine. One of the first books that I read was written by Dr. Richard Mackarness entitled, *Not All in the Mind*[1] that alerted me to the idea that food allergies can have a detrimental impact on both mental and physical health. He suggests that, in evolutionary terms, our bodies are not adjusted to high cereal diets and dairy products, which have only been around for the last few hundred years (it takes thousands of years for our bodies to adjust to evolutionary changes).

He also suggests that up to 80% of the population are probably experiencing some type of food or chemical allergy due to eating highly processed food that our bodies are not yet adjusted to. After reading this book I attempted a detoxification and elimination diet by basically cutting out everything apart from fruit and vegetables.

The first couple of days I felt like my head was going to burst open – the pain and migraines were unbearable, and I spent the weekend in bed sleeping, going to the toilet, and more sleeping. I had mostly vegetable soups, light salads, plenty of fruit and lots of water. On the third day, I awoke feeling so refreshed and alert that I could

---

[1] Mackarness, R. Not All in The Mind. London: Pan Books, 1976.

not believe it! I was hopping around like a little child in a candy store after being imprisoned for so long. The feeling of being alive, pain free and with plenty of energy was amazing!

This renewed energy lasted until the end of the detoxification and elimination diet when I then relapsed back into my old state in a matter of days. What was happening? Why did I feel so good on the detoxification diet, only to find myself back in the prison of pain and misery again after it? Was it related to the food I was eating? Maybe - I was left with more questions than answers.

Unfortunately, I was not as knowledgeable then as I am now. In hindsight, I knew instinctively that something miraculous had happened in my body during the detox, but ignorance could not explain the mechanisms. One of the main reasons I felt so well was because I had simply cut out the foods that I was intolerant to – wheat and dairy – I used to eat cheese sandwiches washed down with coffee most days, as I was too busy to prepare anything else. *"Were these food allergies making me feel so bad?"* I wondered.

Were those unpleasant symptoms I'd experienced in the first couple of days of the detox related to the fact that the stored toxins were being released from my organs and tissues in a big gush?

Again, in retrospect, this is exactly what was happening; during any detoxification regime toxins are released quickly in the first few days, then things slow down somewhat, and the symptoms abate. You begin feeling really well as the body clears itself of accumulated toxins – some of these can be deeply buried in tissues and joints and can cause pain in these areas.

After reading many books on detoxification and experimenting over time, I eventually flew over to England where I saw one of the authors of a nutrition book from the Institute of Optimum Nutrition, Patrick

Holford, and became his student. During the three years of intensive study, I managed to learn a lot that helped my healing process, but not enough to completely heal myself.

My pursuit for learning was intrinsically motivated by my burning desire to completely heal myself. Spanning a 23-year period I studied and obtained degrees and diplomas in Clinical Psychology, Clinical Sexology, Clinical Nutrition, Naturopathy, Herbal Medicine, Homeopathy, Iridology and Su Jok Acupuncture.

I have also studied and trained in numerous diagnostic and therapeutic techniques such as VEGA testing, Bioresonance Therapy, Rife technology, Bach Flower remedies, Thermography, Darkfield Microscopy and Live Blood Analysis, Low Intensity Laser Therapy, Autonomic Response Testing, Field Control Therapy, Biological Terrain Analysis, heavy metal analysis using atomic fluorescence and inductively coupled plasma optical emission spectrometers, as well as many varied detoxification techniques.

Regaining My Health

After these long, interesting years of study I eventually managed to regain my health and optimize it. This year (2016) I am 60 years old and have plenty of energy and the well-being to do all the things that I like doing, including flying a small private plane, horse riding, maintaining antique cars and motorbikes, water skiing, writing books, and researching and running the busy Da Vinci Natural Health Centre[2], of which I am the Founder Director, based in Larnaca, Cyprus. I am also the Founder and Academic Director of the Da Vinci College of Holistic Medicine[3], as well as being involved with many other projects and activities too numerous to mention.

---

[2] www.naturaltherapycenter.com
[3] www.collegenaturalmedicine.com

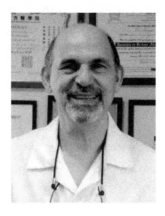

Dr. George J. Georgiou (2018)

My Diverse and Evolving Clinical Practice

While my passion for maintaining my own health has not abated, I have developed a new passion: to help my patients recover their health, just like I did. I always felt disappointed when a patient did not respond well to my treatments.

When some of my patients failed to see any health benefits, I asked myself, *"What could I have done better or different?"* I kept researching and reflecting on the why and the how - I strove to improve and optimize the therapeutic protocols I was offering that could resolve the multitude of problems facing my patients. I began analyzing old and new cases. I researched the literature, tested many new and different therapeutic protocols, refined them or discarded them on the basis of clinical outcomes. When I could not find suitable therapeutic protocols available, I formulated new ones. Those that tested positive were retained; the failed ones were discarded.

My continuous training and research, combined with the feedback from my patients, enabled me to optimize and customize the treatment methodology to the needs of individual patients: *bespoke medicine.* I began observing many of my patients recovering from serious ill-health and eventually experiencing the health transformation that I had personally experienced. In the beginning, I was not so sure; perhaps it was a fluke? Perhaps it was coincidental? Perhaps it was luck?

I was getting some amazing results, but I thought to myself, *"Let us not get carried away. This could be based on some patients coincidentally recovering and not based on my methodology."* But the results were replicable with more and more patients, and with different and varied conditions, even though the treatments differed for each patient having the same disease.

The word spread, and I began getting referrals for more serious cases: chronic degenerative diseases such as arthritis, multiple sclerosis, heart disease, diabetes and cancer – many of them coming in from abroad. These cases were tough and needed special attention. Cancer was a real challenge. How do you approach patients that were literally given a few months to live? I had to stretch my knowledge and experience to new limits. I had to change the whole framework in which I worked. Serious cases required private attention for nearly a whole day. I had to get appropriate equipment, invest in a bigger library. I had no space to put it all, so I built a larger Centre, fully equipped, with in-house laboratory facilities.

While I was active in clinical practice, I also engaged in academic and empirical research – especially on heavy metal toxicity. After three years of arduous research in laboratories and in the field, I developed a unique product called HMD™[4] of which I am now the worldwide patent-pending holder. I have published a number of articles in peer-reviewed journals and I am regularly invited to conferences to talk about my research, clinical methodology, as well as my unique therapeutic protocols.

I have had a rewarding and successful career, blessed with the

---

[4] www.worldwidehealthcenter.net

satisfaction of helping people regain their health and their lives. There is nothing more spiritually rewarding than having a patient who has been given a zero prognosis from the medical fraternity, regain complete health. This in itself is enough to motivate me to work until the day that I die.

Success Breeds Success... and Jealousy

Success breeds success – it also breeds jealousy. My clinical work caused discomfort among the local medical establishment. The "miraculous" natural cures of patients did not resonate well with conventional medicine. I was hounded by the Cyprus Medical Association, constantly being reported to the police and General Attorney for "practicing medicine without being a qualified medical practitioner." I was arrested and handcuffed on one occasion (I spent one evening giving health advice to police jail guards!)

All this was harassment by the "powers that be", all motivated by jealousy, greed, ego and self-interest, not by patients' interests. After all, none of my patients complained to me or reported me for negligence or unprofessionalism – it was always the medical association who would undergo the "witch hunt" using every influence that they could to exterminate those that were getting in their way.

I began getting banned from appearing on TV after talks with the allopathic medical doctors. When I presented patients on TV that had been cured of Crohn's, Irritable Bowel Syndrome, Multiple Sclerosis, cardiovascular problems and more, the powerful lobby of the medical profession made certain I did not appear again.

I also began getting banned from discussing issues of holistic vs allopathic medicine. It appears that the media here in Cyprus is no more democratic or objective with freedom of speech than most of the Illuminati-owned channels abroad. Continuing with this education in

Holistic Medicine would certainly have been beneficial to the viewers and their families, but this was not the issue.

Even though I was hounded on several occasions, I was never convicted even once. The charges were thrown out by the Attorney General even before reaching a court of law - there simply was "no case." Even the police got criticized by the medical fraternity for "not doing their job properly and not being strict enough with charlatans." The harassments continue even now, and so do attempts to lock me away and silence me.

As much as I do not like the reaction and the actions of conventional medics and their associations – I understand them fully. There is a lot at stake, ranging from bruised egos to big money. My treatment methodology is not only effective – it costs a fraction of the money spent on their conventional, ineffective, as well as risky treatments.

The more patients who are treated using Holistic Medicine, the more resistance there is from the medical profession – it's an irony as one would think that they would pay attention. But it is not the motive to heal that is the primary factor, but the gargantuan ego and self-interest.

In Cyprus where I have been working for over 33 years, I have been attacked by the Cyprus Medical Association more times than I care to remember – usually this takes place about every 5 years where I get a call from the police saying that the Cyprus Medical Association is bringing charges against me for "practicing medicine without being a qualified medical practitioner."

The police come around to the Centre with search warrants, take what they want, bully me around and ask a myriad of questions to "catch me out" and take photos of anything that they wish. There is no arguing with them as they normally appear in force, rummaging through my personal desk, taking personal diaries that have no relevance to their case, and generally bullying me to frighten and weaken the "enemy."

These scare tactics do not scare me, but they irritate me. It is an inconvenience and an invasion of privacy, but one has to stand firm and be chivalrous in these matters, as truth and innocence triumph in the end.

I hope I do not bore you with details of my personal journey, but I felt that it would be pertinent to share these experiences with you so that you understand that I came from a place of suffering and persecution, and this has helped me to be more compassionate and empathic with my patients, which is healing in itself.

Now it is time to examine the conceptual aspects of treating Candida, which has a variety of components that are important to follow if one is going to succeed. There are numerous approaches to treating Candida, from medical doctors using pharmaceutical anti-fungal medication, to naturopaths and nutritionists using a variety of natural products to kill off the Candida. All these treatments are rampant with problems that end up in the patient feeling better initially, only to find that the Candida "creeps back" again after a few months.

It took me over 11 years to finally rid myself of Candida, after pursuing many different therapies from experts who had written books on the subject.

I will share with you the secrets that I discovered while formulating the Da Vinci Candida Protocol, that has now been published in peer-reviewed journals[5,6] and has been implemented with over 5,000 patients at the Da Vinci Holistic Health Centre, with astounding success.

CHAPTER 2:
What is Candida?

Every person lives in a virtual sea of microorganisms, (bacteria, viruses, parasites, stealth organisms and fungi). These microbes can reside in the throat, mouth, nose, intestinal tract, almost anywhere; they are as much a part of our bodies as the food we eat. Usually, these microorganisms do not cause illness, unless our resistance becomes lowered.

Candida albicans is yeast that lives in the mouth, throat, intestines and genitourinary tract of most humans. It is usually considered to be a normal part of the bowel flora (the organisms that coexist with us in our lower digestive tract). It is actually a member of a broader classification of organisms known as fungi.

Candida are unicellular yeasts that are somewhat larger than bacteria. They mostly divide asexually and can switch between a yeast and a pseudohyphal or hyphal form. Like other yeasts, Candida flourish in habitats where there is an abundance of sugar.

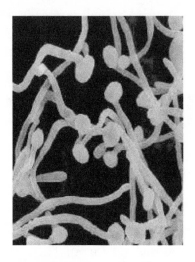

Pathogenic, mycelial Candida

Candida are normal human commensals, particularly in the mouth, skin, vagina and intestine. Candida can be cultured from faeces in up to 80% of healthy adults[7]. Candida numbers increase significantly following antibacterial therapy[8], but the numbers seem to be unaffected by a refined carbohydrate diet[9]. It seems likely that intestinal Candida numbers are regulated in a similar way as intestinal bacteria[10].

The uncontrolled growth of Candida is known as "Candida overgrowth" or "Candidiasis".

Women are more likely to get Candida overgrowth than men. This is related to the female sex hormone 'progesterone', which is elevated in the last half of the menstrual cycle. Progesterone increases the amount of glycogen (animal starch, easily converted to sugar) in the vaginal tissues which provide an ideal growth medium for Candida. Progesterone levels also elevate during pregnancy. Men are affected less frequently but are by no means invulnerable.

C. Albicans and C. glabrata are the two most common Candida species that cause Systemic Candidiasis. There are 81 different types of Candida species such as C. glabrata, krusei, lusitaniae, parapsilosis, tropicalis and more. However, only half a dozen are commonly found in humans, with C. albicans dominating. More than 70% of Candida species found in humans are Candida albicans.

How Do You Get It?

Candida albicans prefers people. Candida enters newborn infants during or shortly after birth. Usually, the growth of the yeast is kept in check by the infant's immune system and thus produces no overt symptoms. But, should the immune response weaken, the condition known as oral thrush can occur. By six months of age, 90% of all babies test positive for Candida and by adulthood, virtually all humans play host to Candida albicans and are thus engaged in a life-long relationship.

Unfortunately, there are many factors in our modern society that can upset the ecological balance of the body, weaken the immune system and allow the yeast to overgrow. Of these, the major risk factors which may predispose one to the proliferation of Candida are:

•STEROID HORMONES, IMMUNOSUPPRESSANT DRUGS such as cortisone, which treat severe allergic problems by paralyzing the immune system's ability to react.

•PREGNANCY, MULTIPLE PREGNANCIES or BIRTH CONTROL PILLS which upset the body's hormonal balance.

•DIETS HIGH IN CARBOHYDRATE AND SUGAR INTAKE, YEAST AND YEAST PRODUCTS, AS WELL AS MOULDS AND FERMENTED FOODS

•PROLONGED EXPOSURE TO ENVIRONMENTAL MOULDS

•ANTIBIOTICS and SULPHA DRUGS - Probably the chief culprit of all. Antibiotics kill all bacteria, they do not distinguish good bacteria from bad. Antibiotics kill the "good" flora which normally keeps the Candida under control. This allows for the unchecked growth of Candida in the intestinal tract. It is normally difficult to recover a yeast culture from bodily surfaces. However, after 48 hours of taking tetracycline, yeast can be cultured easily from anyone.

In the Kaiser Health News report in June 2016, this was what was said against antibiotics and the lethal fungus that can be created (another Candida species known as C. auris):

"Hospitalized patients are at especially high risk from the fungus because many have had antibiotics, which can kill off healthy bacteria that help protect us from disease." Said Peter Hotez, dean of the National School of Tropical Medicine at Baylor College of Medicine in Houston.

"It's a warning or wake-up against the indiscriminate use of antibiotics, especially in hospital settings," Hotez said.

"Hospitals have been testing for the fungus more frequently due to outbreaks in Asia and the United Kingdom", said Amesh Adalja, senior associate at the UPMC Center for Health Security in Baltimore.

"In earlier outbreaks, the fungus has killed 59 percent of patients, including 68 percent of patients whose infection spread to the bloodstream, said Adalja, who published a brief report on the infection Friday. Previous patients have had a median age of 54", Adalja said. The most common underlying medical problem was diabetes, and half of the patients had undergone surgery within 90 days.

Nearly 80 percent of patients had a catheter placed in a major vein in the chest and 61 percent had a urinary catheter.

"Candida auris is a major threat that carries a high mortality," Adalja said.

"Candida fungal species are ubiquitous. ... As we learn more about this species, it will be essential to understand how it spreads in health care facilities and what the best infection control and treatment strategies are."

What is the Role of Candida?

Candida has two parasitic functions:

1. Gobble up any putrefied food matter in our digestive system (mostly caused by improper digestion due to low stomach acid).

2. After we die, Candida acts to decompose the body, feeding off our corpse and returning us to Mother Earth!

When conditions are right, they transform their yeast form into the hyphal, mycelial state, where filament-like roots invade deep into the mucosa in search of nourishment. The mycelia release enzymes such as phospholipase that attack cell membranes of the mucosa, splitting fatty acids, generating free radicals, and causing inflammation in the intestine and other tissues.

Wherever the yeast colonizes they cause symptoms; whether it's an itchy anus or vagina, diarrhea, heartburn or a sore throat. The mycelial forms release *79 different toxic by-products* that damage specific tissues and organs and will determine which symptoms will occur.

These toxins such as aldehyde can also compete with hormone receptor sites and cause hypothyroidism and hypoestrogenism, as well as binding cortisone, progesterone and other hormones for its own use and causing endocrine deficiency states.

How Does Candida Behave?

Candida albicans is the most common cause of Candidiasis in humans, but other species of Candida such as C. tropicalis, C. parapsilosis, C. of krusei and C. glabrata may also be responsible. The pathogenesis disease associated with Candida in humans is driven by a host of factors.

It was shown recently that gluten and gliadin proteins found in wheat might lead to wheat intolerance with its accompanying symptoms and even trigger celiac disease in genetically susceptible people[11]. Furthermore, a placebo-controlled crossover study revealed that dietary yeast may affect the activity of Crohn's disease[12].

Candida produces alcohol and contains glycoproteins which have the potential to stimulate mast cells to release histamine and apparently prostaglandin (PGE2). These are inflammatory substances which could cause IBS-like symptoms[13,14]. Other circumstantial evidence support the theory of yeasts as a trigger for IBS.

Secretory immunoglobulin A (SIgA) is the front line in the defense of mucous membranes, especially in the intestine. At least three different Candida species are able to produce proteases which can degrade Immunoglobulin A causing inflammation[15].

---

[11] Nieuwenhuizen WF, Pieters RH, Knippels LM, Jansen MC, Koppelman GJ. Is Candida albicans a trigger for the onset of coeliac disease? Lancet 2003; 361 :2152–2154.
[12] Barclay GR, McKenzie H, Pennington J, Parratt D, Pennington CR. The effect of dietary yeast on the activity of stable chronic Crohn's disease. Scand J Gastroenterol 1992; 27 :196–200.
[13] Romani L, Bistoni F, Puccetti P. Initiation of T-helper cell immunity to Candida albicans by IL-12: the role of neutrophils. Chem Immunol. 1997; 68:110-35.
[14] Kanda N, Tani K, Enomoto U, Nakai K & Watanabe S. The skin fungus-induced Th1- and Th2-related cytokine, chemokine and prostaglandin E 2 production in peripheral blood mononuclear cells from patients with atopic dermatitis and psoriasis vulgaris. Clinical & Experimental Allergy; 32(8):1243-50.
[15] Reinholdt J, Krogh P, Holmstrup P. Degradation of IgA1, IgA2, and S-IgA by candida and torulopsis species. Acta Path Microbiol Immunol Scand, Sect C 1987; 95:65-74

C. albicans is a diploid organism which has eight sets of chromosome pairs. Interestingly, Candida is one of the few microorganisms that have a diploid gene controlling the same protein – this means that it is capable of changing forms from the normal candida to a more virulent mycelial form that can penetrate and destroy tissues.

When Does Candida Become A Problem?

The problem begins when the normal, budding Candida species that we have in our gut, which 90% of babies are born with, actually changes form to the mycelial or hyphae form which is pathogenic or disease-causing. This only happens when the internal milieu of the gut and other tissues becomes more acidic; either through taking a variety of drugs such as antibiotics that wipes out the friendly flora of the gut, or through eating very acidic foods such as sugar and other refined products.

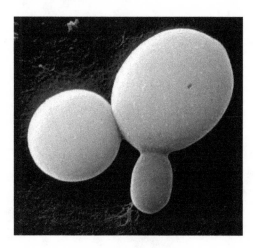

Normal, budding Candida

It appears that this change in pH can trigger genes in the Candida to begin a pleomorphic change into a stealth organism that is very virulent. If fed with sugar, it can increase itself from 1 to 100 cells in 24 hours. These 100 cells can then produce 100 each in the next 24 hours, and so on. So, by the 4th day we will have 100 million Candida cells – this is exponential, explosive growth!

Research has shown that it does not take longer than 1-2 days for this pathogenic form to go deep into the body tissues, inflaming them and damaging them in the process

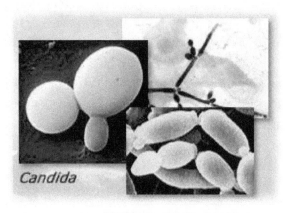

Normal budding Candida on the left, and pathogenic on the right

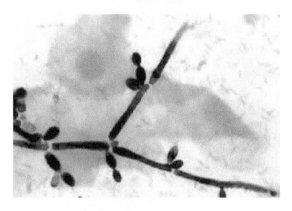

Mycelial, pathogenic form: Pseudohyphae with chlamydospores (grape-like spores) making up the clusters of blastoconidia

How Does Candida Attack the Body?

When candida attacks the body, it does it in various stages. First, the candida adheres to host cells, a bit like glue. Candida binds to the proteins of mucosal or endothelial cells of the host (Calderone, et al, 2001; Grubb et al, 2008).

The close association with cell surfaces stimulates the formation of biofilms (Kumato et al, 2005). The biofilm surrounds the yeast cells like a protective cocoon and wards off attacks from the environment - including the immune system of the host.

These biofilms can also make the candida more resistant to anti-fungal drugs, since they push out these drugs from the cells. There is also reduced production of ergosterol in the cell membrane, which makes the yeast cells less sensitive to anti-fungals by a factor of 30 to 2,000 (Douglas, L.J., 2003).

In addition, C. albicans can secrete 10 different enzymes known collectively as aspartate proteinases (SAPs) which invade the tissues and organs (Hube, B, 2010; Thewes et al, 2007; Polakova et al, 2009).

C. albicans is also able to rapidly change its cell surface structure, making it more difficult for the immune system to recognize these cells. This is known as "phenotypic switching." This process is likely triggered by biofilm formation (Soll, D.R., 2002; Morita, E 1999; Pappas et al, 2004; Reinel et al, 2008).

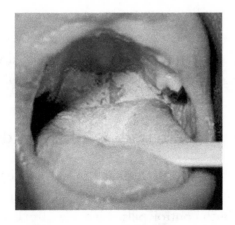

Candida attacking the mouth

21

C. albicans also manages to "trick" the immune system because of its ability to change forms from the normal round yeast cell, to the protracted hyphae form. This results in the beta-glucan molecules in the external wall layers being blocked (Netea et al, 2008). As a consequence, the immune system can no longer recognize the fungi or initiate an immune reaction; they are designed to recognise the beta-glucan of the Candida cell wall (Bastidas et al, 2009; Romani et al, 2003; Berman, J, 2006).

The transition from the yeast to the hyphae form - and back again - is a process known as 'pleomorphism' (the ability to change forms). It is controlled by the synthesis of inflammatory chemicals in the body known as *prostaglandins* (PGE2) and *leukotrienes* (LTB4), (Bastidas et al, 2009; Noverr et al, 2005; Noverr et al, 2004, Noverr et al, 2001; Carlyle et al, 2009).

Pleomorphism is also controlled by contact with bacterial peptidoglycans (Xu et al, 2008). Interestingly, when antibiotics are taken, this leads to the release of peptidoglycans from the cell wall of intestinal bacteria, which increase the production of hyphae from C. albicans, therefore making them more aggressive and more invasive (Pilspanen et al, 2008).

Some Candida strains avoid the attacks of the immune system by concealing themselves in host cells. They can survive unharmed in epithelial cells (Filler et al, 2006) or in non-activated white blood cells called macrophages (Raska et al, 2007; Dalkilic et al, 1991) and even replicate there.

Anyone Can Be Affected with Candida

Anyone can be infected with Candida today! Women can be infected because of antibiotics, steroids, anti-inflammatory medications, hormones and birth-control pills. Men are also being infected with Candida from antibiotics, steroids, anti-inflammatory drugs, pain medications, and sexual relations with an infected partner (even though this often results in a topical infection, not a systemic spread).

Teenagers can get Candida from routine treatment with tetracycline or other antibiotics for acne.

Babies have Candida from the birth canal or breast milk of the infected mother. That is why babies often have thrush (a white-coated tongue), which is a yeast infection.

Millions of people all over the world are infected with Candida. It is estimated that at least 1 in 3 people in the Western world are affected. Because so many of the population can be infected, and because so many factors can cause the condition, Candida is an enormous health problem today.

Candida coexists in our bodies with many species of bacteria in a competitive balance. Other bacteria act to keep Candida growth in check in our body ecology. When we are healthy, the immune system keeps Candida proliferation under control, but when the immune response is weakened, Candida growth can proceed unchecked.

It is an opportunistic organism, one which, when given the opportunity, will attempt to colonize all acidic bodily tissues. This is one of the reasons why it is present in all tumours, since they have a very acidic pH. This uncontrolled growth of Candida is known as "Candida overgrowth" or "Candidiasis".

Fungus with Many Faces

A distinctive characteristic of C. albicans is its ability to grow with three distinct morphologies:

1. Yeast
2. Pseudohyphae
3. True hyphae

See Fig. 1 below that illustrates the difference between these 3 forms. This is the same fungus, but it can change forms when given the right circumstances. This is typically known as PLEOMORPHISM, which is the Greek word for *"many shapes or morphologies"*.

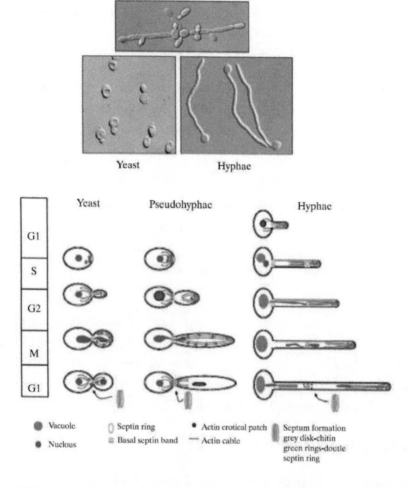

Fig 1. Different growth morphologies of C. albicans (reproduced from Sudbery et al., 2004).

Of all these forms, the Hyphal form is the worst as it can be aggressive and destroy tissues, causing symptoms and diseases. In other words, it is virulent or disease causing.

24

This form of virulent fungus is created when environmental conditions are conducive; such as a 37°C growth temperature, the presence of serum, neutral pH, high CO2, growth in embedded conditions and the presence N-acetylglucosamine.

Figure 3 shows this aggressive, hyphal form of C. albicans, aggressively infiltrating the human small intestine.

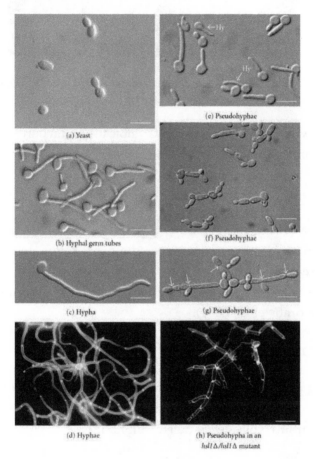

Figure 2: Yeast, hyphal and pseudohyphal (this figure is reproduced with permission from Sudbery et al).

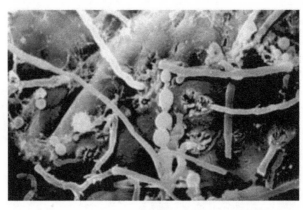

Fig 3. Candida albicans on human small intestine mucosa 3000X (taken by Ms A Lorenz, with kind permission of Ardeypharm GmbH)

The less virulent yeast form of C. albicans is favoured by a 30°C growth temperature and acidic pH (pH 4.0). Pseudohyphal growth is really an intermediate, transitional stage between the yeast form (less virulent) to the most virulent hyphal form. This can occur in temperatures of 35°C or a pH of 5.5.

Formation of hyphae from yeast mother cells is regulated by a quorum-sensing mechanism in which yeast cells produce small molecules, such as the alcohol farnesol, that inhibit the formation of hyphae (Hornby et al., 2001).

Biofilms

Have you ever picked up a rock from a nearby stream and wondered why it's slimy on the surface? That slimy layer is actually a group of microorganisms, collectively called a biofilm.

A biofilm is a community of bacteria that attach to a surface by excreting a sticky, sugary substance that encompasses the bacteria in a matrix. This might be the first time you've heard the term biofilm, but they're all around us; in streams, drains, fish tanks, even on our teeth.

A biofilm can be composed of a single species or a conglomerate of species. In many cases, biofilms are only bacteria, but they can also include other living things such as fungi and algae, creating a microbial stew of sorts. Biofilms are complex systems that are sometimes compared to multicellular organisms.

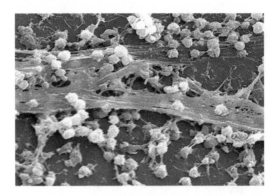

Biofilm of Candida

C. albicans is able to form a biofilm that basically protects it from being attacked by the immune system of the host (Blankenship and Mitchell, 2006; Nobile and Mitchell, 2006).

This biofilm of Candida is composed of proteins, carbohydrates, fibrinogen or fibrin, and polynucleotides that contain RNA and DNA material. This structure is bound together with ligands that are extremely sticky.

As we will see later, the Enlyse™ enzymes present in one of the remedies used for treating Candida – CANDA PLUS - can eradicate this biofilm, hence allowing the immune system to do its work.

Symptoms Related to Candida

There are many symptoms that can be caused by Candida – here is a list by Dr. Jeff Mc Comb's, D.C., a chiropractor working in the U.S. who has also created a Candida Library with hundreds of research papers on Candida: http://www.candidalibrary.org/cand_lib/

This is a list of 100 Common Candida Symptoms associated with systemic fungal candida from his website:

* ADD
* ADHD
* Acid reflux
* Acne
* Allergies
* Anxiety
* Arthritis
* Asthma
* Athlete's foot
* Autism
* Autoimmune conditions
* Bladder infections
* Blisters in mouth
* Bloating
* Blood sugar imbalances
* Body odour
* BPH
* Brain fog
* Bronchitis
* Burping
* Cancer
* Chemical sensitivities
* Chronic Fatigue Syndrome
* Colitis
* Concentration difficulty
* Confusion
* Congestion
* Constipation
* Crohn's Disease
* Cough
* Cystitis
* Depression

* Dermatitis
* Diabetes
* Diarrhoea
* Eczema
* Endometriosis
* Excess mucous
* Fibromyalgia
* Flatulence
* Fluid retention
* Food allergies
* Food cravings
* Frequent colds
* Frequent infections
* Fungal infections
* Gas
* Gastritis
* Genital rashes
* Headaches
* Heartburn * Hormonal imbalances
* Hypoglycaemia
* Hypothyroidism
* Irritability
* Inflammatory Bowel Disease (IBD / IBS)
* Immune system dysfunction
* Impotence
* Indigestion
* Infertility
* Irregular menstruation
* Itchy skin
* Joint pain
* Lack of mental clarity
* Leaky gut
* Lethargy
* Lupus

* Migraines
* Memory problems
* Mood swings
* Muscle pain
* Nail fungus
* Osteoarthritis
* Penile itching
* PMS
* Poor concentration
* Poor memory
* Prostatitis
* Prostate enlargement
* Psoriasis
* Rashes
* Rectal itching
* Rheumatoid arthritis
* Rhinitis
* Scleroderma
* Sexual dysfunction
* Sinus problems
* Sores
* Sore throat
* Sugar cravings
* Swollen joints
* Thrush
* Urethritis
* Urinary frequency
* Vaginal infections
* Vaginitis
* Visual problems
* Weakness
* Weight gain
* White coating on tongue

What are the Signs of Candida Infection?

The result of heightened Candida overgrowth is a list of adverse symptoms of considerable length. But basically, the characteristics of Candida overgrowth fall under three categories, those affecting:

1. The gastrointestinal and genitourinary tracts

2. Allergic responses

3. Mental/emotional manifestations

Initially the signs will show near the sights of the original yeast colonies. Most often the first signs are seen in conditions such as nasal congestion and discharge, nasal itching, blisters in the mouth, sore or dry throat, abdominal pain, belching, bloating, heartburn, constipation, diarrhea, rectal burning or itching, vaginal discharge, vaginal itching or burning, increasingly worsening symptoms of PMS, prostatitis, impotence, frequent urination, burning on urination, bladder infections.

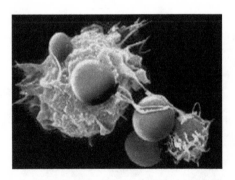

White blood cell killing Candida

But, if the immune system remains weak for long enough, Candida can spread to all parts of the body causing an additional plethora of problems, such as fatigue, drowsiness, incoordination, lack of concentration, mood swings, dizziness, headaches, bad breath, coughing, wheezing, joint swelling, arthritis, failing vision, spots in front of the eyes, ear pain, deafness, burning or tearing eyes, muscle aches, depression, irritability, sweet cravings, increasing food and chemical sensitivities, numbness and tingling, cold hands and feet, asthma, hay fever, multiple allergies, hives and rashes, eczema, psoriasis, chronic fungal infections like athlete's foot, ringworm and fingernail/toenail infections.

In addition, **79 different toxic products** are released by Candida, which in itself places a considerable burden on the immune system. These get into the bloodstream and travel to all parts of the body where they may give rise to a host of adverse symptoms. Yeasts in the body produce a by-product called acetaldehyde, a toxic substance resulting in several health consequences. In fact, acetaldehyde is the compound that produces the symptoms in an alcohol "hang-over."

In Candida overgrowth, the yeast colonies can dig deep into intestinal walls, damaging the bowel wall in their colonization. The invasive Candida filaments produce disease affecting the entire body in a number of ways...

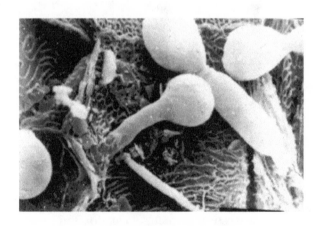

Candida penetrating human tissue

Destruction of the intestinal membrane, allowing for:

•Severe leaks of toxins from undesirable microorganisms within the layers of encrusted fecal matter into the bloodstream causing a variety of symptoms and aggravating many pre-existing conditions. Under the anaerobic conditions of the colon, Candida itself will produce a number of toxins by fermenting sugars.

•Absorption of incompletely digested dietary proteins. These are extremely allergenic and may produce a large spectrum of allergic reactions. Food allergies are very common with Candidiasis, as is environmental hypersensitivity (to smoke, auto exhaust, natural gas, perfumes, air pollutants), probably due to Candida filaments infiltrating lung and sinus membranes.

•Migration of Candida itself into the bloodstream. Once in the blood, it has access to all body tissues and may cause various gland or organ dysfunctions, weakening the entire system and further lowering resistance to other diseases

Candida can also attack the immune system, causing suppressor cell disease, in which the immune system produces antibodies to everything at the slightest provocation, resulting in extreme sensitivities.

Finally, Candida overgrowth can be dangerous if not controlled. The persistent, constant challenge to the immune system by an ever-increasing, long-term overgrowth of Candida can eventually serve to wear down the immune system and cause a seriously weakened capacity for resistance to disease.

How is Candida Diagnosed?

The patient's history and symptoms are usually the key to arriving at a diagnosis. There are a wide variety of signs and symptoms that are prevalent in Systemic Candidiasis; being able to score these systematically provides a good, overall picture.

Dr. Crook, an American trained medical doctor and lecturer, after repeated observations of his patients became interested in chronic health complaints related to yeast overgrowth and the related nutritional and environmental factors.

Dr. Crook was one of the modern-day pioneers who published the book, *The Yeast Connection*, and brought the concept of yeast infections to the public eye, while also trying to teach his colleagues, which was not easy at the best of times. In this book, he developed a comprehensive questionnaire of many of the symptoms that are related to systemic Candidiasis.

Dr. Crook's Candida questionnaire (see Appendix) enables the patient to score their symptoms and arrive at a number. Anything above 180 for women and 140 for men is highly significant and represents the majority of symptoms that relate to Candida infestation.

There are cases, however, that may still have the pathological form of Candida, but score low on this questionnaire, so other tests are required to confirm the diagnosis.

There are also other testing procedures for picking up on the Candida; the Vegetative Reflex Testing (VRT), biodermal screening, a form of Bioresonance testing initially invented by Dr. Voll and later adapted by Dr Schimmel.

In the case of identifying the pathological, hyphal form of Candida, as long as the practitioner has an ampoule of this form, then it is very easy to test whether the patient is resonating to it. In the hands of an experienced practitioner, this is an accurate and efficient way of testing, given that there are no real clinical tests for pathological Candida that have been developed yet, short of taking a biopsy from specific organs and tissues of the body.

There are a number of Bioresonance testing devices; the VEGA, the BICOM, the DETA PROFESSIONAL and more. Practitioners choose the one that they can afford, but perhaps the most cost effective device is the DETA PROFESSIONAL (http://www.deta-elis-uk.com).

I run 5-day intensive clinical workshops 3-4 times per year training practitioners to use VRT bioresonance testing and treatment in Larnaca, Cyprus. There is also an online course to help practitioners understand the theory entitled, *Energy Medicine and Bioresonance.* (http://www.collegenaturalmedicine.com).

Another method of testing the Candida is to use a form of kinesiological muscle testing called Autonomic Response Testing (ART) invented by a German neurologist, Dr. Dietrich Klinghardt, M.D. Ph.D. ART grew out of the importance of detecting and correct problems of the autonomic nervous system (ANS).

ART allows the practitioner to correct the problems of the ANS and to help restore the self-regulating mechanism of the body, allowing the patient to return to a state of health.

To date, there is no conclusive blood or clinical test for diagnosing pathogenic Systemic Candidiasis. There are expensive genetic tests that can determine the genome of the mycelial, hyphal, pathogenic Candida, but these are not generally available on the open market as of yet and are used more for research purposes.

Laboratory Tests

Laboratory tests have their advantages and disadvantages – let's take a look at some of them:

An easy-to-use diagnostics platform rapidly identifies *Candida* yeast species directly from positive blood cultures. The new assay, peptide nucleic acid fluorescence in situ hybridization (PNA FISH), is a highly sensitive and specific assay that uses PNA probes to target species-specific ribosomal RNA (rRNA) in bacteria and yeasts.

Called the Yeast Traffic Light, the assay is one of the latest molecular-based PNA FISH diagnostic platforms that provides rapid identification of bloodstream pathogens in hours instead of days. Laboratories can identify, in a single Yeast Traffic Light test, up to five Candida species directly from positive blood cultures, including C. *albicans* and/or C. *parapsilosis*, C. *tropicalis*, and C. *glabrata* and/or C. *krusei*, enabling clinicians to provide early, effective and appropriate antifungal therapy for patients afflicted with Candidemia.

The results of the test indicate the yeast responsible for the infection; green fluorescing cells indicate C. *albicans* and/or C. *parapsilosis*; yellow fluorescing cells indicate C. *tropicalis*; and red fluorescing cells are C. *glabrata* and/or C. *krusei*.

Other laboratory tests are also available, but none are completely accurate at identifying the pathological, mycelial form of Candida.

Antibiotic Abuse and Inappropriate Prescribing

The prevalence of Candida today may be most directly related to the widespread societal exposure to antibiotics. From prescriptions for colds, infections, acne, and from additional consumption of antibiotic-treated foods such as meats, dairy, poultry and eggs.

Notably, antibiotics do not kill viruses; they only destroy bacteria. Yet, they are universally prescribed for all colds, flus and other viral problems. Such indiscriminate and extensive use of antibiotics is not only considered a primary cause of Candida overgrowth but is recently being found to be responsible for the unbridled development of "killer bacteria."

The rapid and direct proliferation of the yeast following antibiotic use strongly suggests that the problem of Candida is one which stems from an inner state of imbalance, rather than from an outside attack by a microbe or disease. This is a very important point to understand if one wishes to get rid of an overgrowth problem, because it suggests that

Candida is not so much a problem as is the body's own failure to control it!

☐ Incorrectly prescribed antibiotics also contribute to the promotion of resistant bacteria (Center for Disease Control and Prevention).

☐ Studies have shown that treatment type, choice of agent, or duration of antibiotic therapy is incorrect in 30% to 50% of cases (Luyt, C.E, 2014).

☐ One U.S. study reported that a pathogen was defined in only 7.6% of 17,435 patients hospitalized with community-acquired pneumonia (CAP) (Barlett, J.G., 2013).

☐ In comparison, investigators at the Karolinska Institute in Sweden were able to identify the probable pathogen in 89% of patients with CAP through use of molecular diagnostic techniques. Therefore, prescribing the correct antibiotics for this particular health problem, as opposed to experimenting with many different types, to the detriment of the patient.

☐ 30% to 60% of the antibiotics prescribed in intensive care units (ICUs) have been found to be unnecessary, inappropriate, or suboptimal (Luyt, C.E., 2014).

☐ Incorrectly prescribed antibiotics have questionable therapeutic benefit and expose patients to potential complications of antibiotic therapy (Lushniak, B.D., 2014).

☐ Sub-inhibitory and sub-therapeutic antibiotic concentrations can promote the development of antibiotic resistance by supporting genetic alterations, such as changes in gene expression, HGT, and mutagenesis (Viswanathan, V.K.,2014).

Why Is It A Serious Problem?

Once begun, if not recognized and treated appropriately, Candida overgrowth can result in a self-perpetuating, negative cycle. Large numbers of yeast germs can weaken the immune system, which normally protects the body from harmful invaders. Even though Candida is part of the ecological balance in the body since birth, it is still recognized by the immune system as a foreign body that needs to be controlled.

So, when overgrowth occurs, a chronic stimulation to the immune system results - every second, every minute, every hour, every day, every month, every year - in an attempt by the immune system to regain control. In time, it is believed that this can exhaust the immune system, predisposing one to more serious degenerative diseases. Many believe chronic drains on the immune system such as Candida and parasites can play a direct role in the development of cancer and AIDS. Seen in this light, Candida overgrowth should not be taken lightly.

Candida produces its effects by two routes. Firstly, there is a direct route initially by invasion of the gut and the vagina; Candida is capable of spreading along the entire length of the gut. The presence of chronic vaginitis can often indicate wide-spread Candidiasis. Secondly, there can be indirect effects caused by the spread of mycotoxins through the bloodstream to other sites.

In the gut, Candida can alter its form from a simple yeast organism to a "mycelial fungal form" with a network of root-like fibres called rhizoids. These can penetrate and damage the gut lining, allowing foreign food proteins to be absorbed into the bloodstream and to challenge the immune system so that multiple food allergies or intolerances may result.

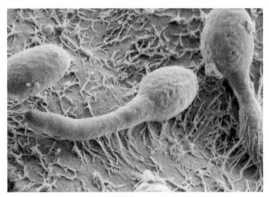

Electron micrograph of C. albicans

Toxic waste from Candida can also be absorbed into the bloodstream causing "Yeast Toxin Hypersensitivity". This leads to symptoms such as anxiety, depression and impaired intellectual functioning. The main toxin implicated here is acetaldehyde, which is a normal by-product of metabolism, produced in small amounts and rendered harmless by the liver.

If, however, there is excess production of this by Candida, particularly in low-oxygen environments, and a lack of the appropriate liver enzymes which tend to be deficient in 5% of the general population, the acetaldehyde will become bound strongly to human tissue. This may cause impaired neuro-transmission in the brain resulting in anxiety, depression, defective memory and cloudy thinking.

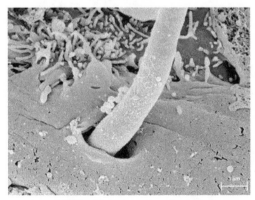

Rhizoid penetrating tissue

Acetaldehyde, one of the mycotoxins secreted by Candida, is responsible for a large part of the cellular damage that occurs. Acetaldehyde in the intestinal wall and liver will upset absorption through the intestine, as well as impairing the function of white blood cells (lymphocytes) and red blood cells.

In order to break down these nasty mycotoxins, adequate amounts of glutamine, selenium, niacin, folic acid, B6, B12, iron, and molybdenum are required. Certainly, patients exhibiting toxic syndrome while treating Candida are highly recommended to take these food supplements for their own protection.

[16] Iwata, K.; Yamamoto, Y "Glycoprotein Toxins Produced by Candida albicans." Proceedings of the Fourth International Conference on the Mycoses, PAHO Scientific Publication #356, June 1977.

CHAPTER 3:

The Relationship Between Candida and Chronic Diseases

Several natural medicine practitioners have long been supporting the notion that intestinal fungi can contribute to chronic diseases.

However, the allopathic medical fraternity has been downplaying the role of intestinal fungi. This is largely since little research has been done; it's difficult to diagnose and it can't be treated properly with pharmaceuticals.

New research at Cedars-Sinai Medical Center looked at the connection between fungi and Ulcerative Colitis.

Dr. David M. Underhill and his team at the *Inflammatory Bowel and Immunobiology Research Institute* have been studying the interaction between Commensal Fungi and the C-Type Lectin Receptor, Dectin-1. In healthy animals, Dectin-1 is produced and works as the body's immune response against fungi.

The risk of developing Ulcerative Colitis increases significantly in mice with a defective form of Dectin-1. Dr. Underhill and his team treated these animals with an antifungal drug called Fluconazole and observed that their symptoms moderated.

---

[16] Iwata, K.; Yamamoto, Y "Glycoprotein Toxins Produced by Candida albicans." Proceedings of the Fourth International Conference on the Mycoses, PAHO Scientific Publication #356, June 1977.

In humans, a mutated form of Dectin-1 is closely related to Ulcerative Colitis that doesn't respond to medical therapy. When this important receptor isn't working properly, our protection against intestinal fungi is decreased and we are more prone to develop Candidiasis.

It's already known that gut flora in patients with UC differs significantly from healthy individuals. The fungal colonization of the colon may influence the activation of UC, and antifungal treatment causes clinical improvement in most individuals. Patients with Crohn's disease and their healthy relatives are colonized with C. albicans more commonly than control families.

30 years after *The Missing Diagnosis* by Orian Truss and *The Yeast Connection* by William Crook were released, there's growing research in the medical community on the importance of gut flora and intestinal fungi.

Candida has also been correlated with chronic inflammatory diseases such as arthritis and multiple sclerosis. That was the implication of a 2012 study in the prestigious journal Nature, conducted by researchers from Charite - Universitatsmedizin Berlin and the Institute for Research in Biomedicine, Bellinzona, Switzerland.

The study found that cells of the fungus Candida albicans seemed to trigger the immune system to produce more inflammation.

The findings are particularly significant because the immune cells being studied play a key role in autoimmune diseases such as multiple sclerosis, rheumatoid arthritis and psoriasis.

"This not only demonstrates that the composition of our microflora has a decisive role in the development of chronic illnesses, but also that the key cells causing illness can develop an anti-inflammatory 'twin'," first author Dr. Christina Zielinski said.

---

[16] Iwata, K.; Yamamoto, Y "Glycoprotein Toxins Produced by Candida albicans." Proceedings of the Fourth International Conference on the Mycoses, PAHO Scientific Publication #356, June 1977.

Effects on Immunity

40 to 60% of all the immune cells in our body are in the gut. The immune system may concurrently also be adversely affected by poor nutrition, heavy exposure to molds in the air, as well as an increasing number of chemicals in our food, water and air, including petrochemicals, formaldehyde, perfumes, cleaning fluids, insecticides, tobacco and other indoor and outdoor pollutants.

Over 10,000 chemicals have been added to our food supplies alone that were not there just 100 years ago! We do not have the genetic recognition of these substances as foods or as useful additions to our bodies.

Specifically, yeast tend to secrete a toxin called Gliotoxin[16] which can disrupt the immune system by inactivating enzyme systems, producing free radicals, which interferes with the DNA of leukocytes and is cytotoxic.

This lowered resistance may not only cause an overall sense of ill-health, but also may allow for the development of respiratory, digestive and other systemic symptoms. One may also become predisposed to developing sensitivities to foods and chemicals in the environment. Such "allergies" may in turn cause the membranes of the nose, throat, ear, bladder and intestinal tract to swell and develop infection.

---

[16] Iwata, K.; Yamamoto, Y "Glycoprotein Toxins Produced by Candida albicans." Proceedings of the Fourth International Conference on the Mycoses, PAHO Scientific Publication #356, June 1977.

Such "allergies" may in turn cause the membranes of the nose, throat, ear, bladder and intestinal tract to swell and develop infection.

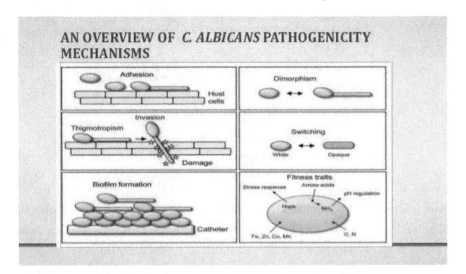

Such conditions may lead the physician to prescribe a "broad spectrum" antibiotic. which may then further promote the overgrowth of Candida and strengthen the existing negative chain of events, leading to further stress on the immune system and increased Candida-related problems.

I have seen this happen in clinical practice many times. If only physicians could think laterally for a minute, many hundreds of thousands of superfluous antibiotic prescriptions could be done away with to the benefit of the patient as opposed to the pharmaceutical industry. Physicians talk about evidence-based medicine, but often drugs such as antibiotics are prescribed for the wrong infections because *testing was not done in the first place.*

The diagram below (Fig 5) clearly shows how Candida is known to impair immune functioning by directly and negatively impacting the helper-suppresser ratio of T lymphocytes.

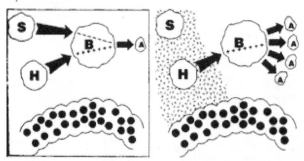

Fig 5: How Yeast Toxins Injure the Immune System
S = Suppressor cell; H = Helper cell; B = B-cell
S=Suppressor cell; H=Helper cell; B=B-cell; A=Antibodies

First diagram: Yeast and intestinal lactobacilli bacteria in balance = normal immune function. A balance between intestinal lactobacilli bacteria and yeast allow for normal immune lymphocyte function. Helper cells stimulate the B-cells to make antibodies, whereas suppressor cells appropriately oppose B-cell antibody production. Antibody production is in balance.

Second diagram: Overgrowth of intestinal yeast, release of toxins into the bloodstream, and altered immune function. Intestinal yeast overgrowth and yeast toxins released into the bloodstream inhibit suppressor cell function. Stimulation of antibody production by helper cells is now unopposed, and inappropriate antibody production occurs. Here we have a heightened state of allergy, as well as an increased susceptibility to autoimmune conditions.

The main components of the immune system are:

1.B-lymphocytes: these produce proteins called immunoglobulins, which bind antigenic substances and render them harmless. An antigen is a substance which the body recognizes as being alien and therefore potentially harmful. An immunoglobulin is a particular kind of protein which coats the antigen; by being made harmless, the antigens can then be digested by other cells.

2. **T-lymphocytes**; there are three types:

a. The killer cells; these attack and destroy substances with enzymes and hormones.

b. The helper cells; these help B cells to make the immunoglobulins.

c. The suppressor cells; these protect the body from the excesses of the body's defense system.

T-cell efficiency can be influenced by nutrition. It is largely the suppressors which are involved in fighting the Candida challenge, partly because Candida's adaptability allows it to produce disguising antigens which deter the immune system from recognizing it as foreign and harmful. In this way, the immune system may eventually become non-responsive to the presence of Candida albicans. Candida toxins will then circulate virtually unchallenged, and Candida will grow in a range of tissues either as a yeast or a mycelial fungus.

This apparent tolerance of Candida by the immune system can only be reversed in the long term by ending exposure of the body to yeast antigens and toxins. A high percentage of serum from symptomless people has been found to contain yeast toxin immunoglobulins. This indicates that the B-cell immune defenses must be constantly counteracting Candida toxin. When alive, yeasts are able to invade the immune system to a certain degree.

When yeast cells are rapidly killed, a die-off (or Herxheimer reaction) occurs and metabolic by-products are released into the body. The Candida yeast cells release 79 different toxins when they die, including ethanol and acetaldehyde.

Here is a list of some of the symptoms you might experience during a die-off (otherwise known as a Herxheimer reaction):

• Nausea
• Headache, fatigue, dizziness

• Swollen glands
• Bloating, gas, constipation or diarrhea
• Increased joint or muscle pain
• Elevated heart rate
• Chills, cold feeling in your extremities
• Body itchiness, hives or rashes
• Sweating
• Fever
• Skin breakouts
• Recurring vaginal, prostate and sinus infections

Other Factors Creating Pathogenesis

The pathogenesis of disease associated with Candida in humans is driven by a multitude of factors. Some strains of candida produce gliotoxin, which may impair neutrophil function. However, candida is a polyantigenic organism containing up to 178 different antigens, which might explain the number of cross-reactions to yeasts, moulds and even human tissue.

It was shown recently that there is a potential cross reactivity with gluten because of several amino acid sequences that are highly homologous to alpha-gliadin and gamma-gliadin. Such a mechanism might lead to wheat intolerance with its accompanying symptoms, and even trigger Celiac disease in genetically susceptible people. Furthermore, a placebo-controlled crossover study has revealed that dietary yeast may affect the activity of Crohn's disease.

Candida produces alcohol and contains glycoproteins, which have the potential to stimulate mast cells to release histamine, and apparently, prostaglandin-inflammatory substances which could cause IBS-like symptoms.

Candida is sensitive to a number of antifungal agents, such as Nystatin, which is not absorbed from the gastrointestinal tract after oral administration. It destroys Candida by binding to sterols in the cell membrane, and thereby increasing permeability with loss of cellular contents.

When other health conditions become involved, Candida becomes known as Candida-related complex (CRC). An excess of Candida in your system can cause a host of uncomfortable signs and symptoms which are syndromes within themselves, such as chronic fatigue syndrome, hypoglycaemia, leaky gut syndrome, fibromyalgia, allergy or sensitivity, hormonal, thyroid, and adrenal dysfunction.

This syndrome isn't caused by the Candida present in our mucosal tissues that cause irritation, inflammation, itchiness, redness and pain, but by the number of metabolites yeast colonies release inside the human colon when they exceed tolerable amounts.

Patients with CRC often have widespread symptoms affecting multiple organs systems such as:

• Gastrointestinal symptoms

• Chronic allergies

• Unexplained fatigue; always tired

• CNS fog, mood swings, depression

• Skin rashes, fungal infections

• Cravings for sugar, bread, beer

Toxicity in the colon affects the health of the whole body, particularly if one's elimination is slowed – like with constipation - due to an imbalance in intestinal flora.

The delicate hormonal and chemical balance that orchestrates our emotional health can also be affected causing symptoms of mental illness.

The Scientific Research on Candida

As we have previously mentioned, there are over 54,000 research articles on Candida on the medical database, PubMed. It is, off course, impossible to do this research justice in a small book of this nature, but let us take a glimpse at some of this scientific research.

The recent research indicates that yeast overgrowth in the intestines does occur and is associated with a variety of symptoms which improve with antifungal treatment. I will quote the scientific references of this research for those that want to look deeper into the topic.

Candida overgrowth of the GI tract was found in recent studies to:

• Promote the development of food allergies by increasing intestinal permeability and affecting immune function. (Gut. 2006 Jul;55(7):954-60; Biosci Microbiota Food Health. 2012;31(4):77-84).

• Aggravate inflammation not only in the gut but in tissues all throughout the body, increasing the risk of allergies and autoimmune diseases. (Med Mycol. 2011 Apr;49(3):237-47; Curr Opin Microbiol. 2011 Aug;14(4):386-91).

• Directly correlate with the amount of inflammation and severity of symptoms in patients with ulcers, Crohn's disease, and ulcerative colitis (J Clin Gastroenterol. 2014 Jul;48(6):513-23; J Physiol Pharmacol. 2009 Mar;60(1):107-18; Curr Opin Microbiol. 2011 Aug;14(4):386-91.

• Increase with the use of antibiotics, especially when there is already inflammation in the intestines (Curr Opin Microbiol. 2011 Aug;14(4):386-91).

• Increase with the use of proton pump inhibitors, otherwise known as anti-acids – drugs that block the production of hydrochloric acid in the stomach (Aliment Pharmacol Ther. 2013 Jun;37(11):1103-11).

• Cause the same symptoms as small intestinal bacterial overgrowth (SIBO) when it occurs in the small intestine (Aliment Pharmacol Ther. 2013 Jun;37(11):1103-11). SIBO symptoms include abdominal pain, chest pain, belching, bloating, fullness, indigestion, nausea, diarrhoea, vomiting, gas, malabsorption, and vitamin deficiencies.

• Promote inflammation in the lungs (Cell Host Microbe. 2014 Jan 15;15(1):95-102).

• Occur more commonly in people with psoriasis and other inflammatory skin disorders (Int J Dermatol. 2014 Dec; 53(12): e555-60.).

•Occur more commonly in people with chronic fatigue syndrome (Scan J Gastro. 2007;42(12):1514-1515.).

•Furthermore, people with irritable bowel syndrome (IBS) have more antibodies in their blood to Candida albicans. The severity of IBS symptoms is directly associated with levels of those antibodies (BMC Gastroenterol. 2012; 12: 166).

•People with "medically unexplained symptoms" who also score highly on a standardized Candida questionnaire called the Fungus Related Disease Questionnaire-7 also have higher levels of antibodies against Candida albicans. These people often have a history of frequent or long-term antibiotic use along with symptoms like frequent yeast infections, sugar cravings, and fatigue (J Altern Complement Med. 2007 Dec;13(10):1129-33). Higher levels of antibodies against Candida albicans indicates the immune system is hypersensitive to the yeast or may simply reflect greater exposure to it (due to Candida yeast overgrowth) (BMC Gastroenterol. 2012; 12: 166.).

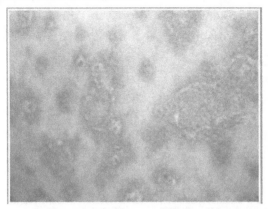

Close-up of rash caused by Candida

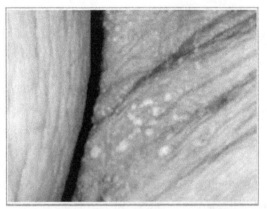

Inflammatory Candida-causing pustules

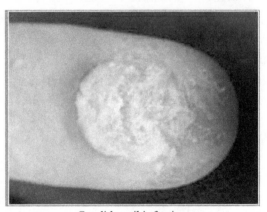

Candida nail infection

Microbial Balance Protects Your Health

This is not the first time that the billions of microorganisms (microbiome) that naturally inhabit the human body, particularly the skin and gut – have been linked to immune system regulation and the prevention or development of autoimmune diseases.

A healthy microbiome also plays a key role in regulating the digestive, nervous and endocrine (hormonal) systems. It even seems to affect mood.

The Candida connection with allergies, asthma, and dermatitis has long been accepted. Current research suggests Candida antigens may trigger celiac and Crohn's disease. Even though these links of Candida to disease are acknowledged, the conventional medical community is hesitant to understand and accept the role of Candida in patients with multiple complaints, often labelled as either non-specific autoimmune disease or more often as psychosomatic illness.

These symptoms include fatigue, muscle pain, joint pain, rashes, dysuria, urinary frequency, vaginitis, and more. Nor do they realize Candida is so often the underlying cause for chronic fatigue syndrome, fibromyalgia, irritable bowel syndrome, environmental exposure syndrome, and central sensitization syndrome.

Candida even effects the brain and can be the precursor to many different mental illnesses from depression to schizophrenia. In other words, when the immune system goes belly up, Candida is almost always a major factor, and yet this connection is often overlooked or ignored.

CHAPTER 4:

Preparing for the Da Vinci Candida Treatment Protocol

I developed the Da Vinci Protocol over many years of study, as well as trial and error with many patients that agreed to experiment – I continue to bow to these patients who helped my learning experience.

Given that we have successfully treated over *5,000 patients* with Candida to date at the Da Vinci Center in Larnaca, Cyprus.

I had spent over 11 years trying to treat my systemic Candidiasis which was causing me many health problems and symptoms including chronic fatigue, brain fog, severe digestive disturbances, fibromyalgia, achlorhydria, pancreatic enzyme deficiencies, concentration and mood disturbances – all these I have already mentioned above.

Before implementing the Da Vinci Candida Protocol with my patients, I make certain that the rest of the body's physiological systems are as optimized as possible.

I generally check for:

1. Food intolerances – these foods are probably one of the biggest sources of internal inflammation and can be a big burden when eradicating the Candida, so it is important to make certain that the patient avoids these foods. I used VRT Bioresonance testing, that I have already discussed, to test over 100 different foods. We will talk more about the mechanisms of food intolerances a little later.

2. Checking for nutritional deficiencies and heavy metals using a Tissue Hair Mineral Analysis test – this involves taking a small sample of hair and sending it to a laboratory abroad.

3. Also, check using Kinesiology, Autonomic Response Testing, Bioresonance Testing, or any other similar test, the status of the stomach and pancreas – usually you will find many patients will not be secreting enough hydrochloric acid from the stomach and enough pancreatic enzymes from the pancreas. So, giving these two in supplement forms is highly recommended to avoid undigested food causing putrefaction in the stomach and gut. I use BETAINE COMPLEX for the stomach and DIGEST PLUS for the gut digestion.

Here is a table summarizing these preparatory steps:

PREPARATION STEPS BEFORE CANDIDA PROTOCOL

TASK	Supplements needed	Comments
1. Food Intolerance test		See a Bioresonance practitioner
2. Hair test for Mineral deficiencies/Heavy metal profile	Supplement what is needed with HMD™ heavy metal detox	Visit: www.worldwideahealthcenter.net
3. Heavy metal detox	Take HMD™, LAVAGE, CHLORELLA	www.worldwidehealthcenter.net
4. Constipated?	Take CONSTFORM and OXYGUT, COLFORM	Visit: www.worldwidehealthcenter.net
5. Digestive issues?	Take DIGESTIZYME & GASTRIC AID	Visit: www.worldwidehealthcenter.net
6. Bioresonance devices	DEVITA AP, DEVITA RITM, DEINFO USB	Visit: www.deta-elis-uk.com
Begin Candida protocol	KANDIDAPLEX, KOLOREX, CAPRYLIC ACID, ACIDOPHILUS & BIFIDUS, CANDIDA 30C	Visit: www.worldwidehealthcenter.net

Tissue Hair Mineral Analysis

In clinical work, I have found one test that I use often, and find to be invaluable - the Hair Tissue Mineral Analysis (HTMA)[17]. This involves taking a small sample of hair by cutting the first inch-and-a-half of growth closest to the scalp at the nape of the neck, or even pubic hair if someone is completely bald. It is then sent to a licensed clinical laboratory where the hair is prepared through a series of chemical and high temperature digestive procedures and is finally analyzed for levels of minerals and toxic metals, by using sophisticated measuring devices called spectrometers.

Hair is considered an ideal tissue for sampling and testing[18]. Firstly, it can be cut easily and painlessly and can be sent to the lab without special handling requirements. Secondly, clinical results have shown that a correctly obtained sample can give an indication of mineral status and toxic metal accumulation following long-term or even acute exposure. Hair is used as one of the tissues of choice by the US Environmental Protection Agency in determining toxic metal exposure. Indeed, several studies have concluded that human hair may be a more appropriate tissue than blood or urine for studying a community's exposure to harmful trace elements.

Although our aim is to rid the body of harmful toxic metals, conversely trace minerals are essential in countless metabolic functions in all phases of the life process[19]. For example, zinc is involved in the production, storage, and secretion of insulin and is necessary for growth hormones. Magnesium is required for normal muscular function, especially the heart. A deficiency in magnesium has been associated with an increased incidence of heart attacks; anxiety and

---

[17] Bland, J. Hair tissue mineral analysis. an emergent diagnostic technique. Thorsons Publishers, USA, 1983.
[18] Watts, DL. Trace Elements and Other Essential Nutrients: Clinical Application of Tissue Mineral Analysis.
[19] Wilson, LD. Nutritional Balancing and Hair Mineral Analysis: A Comprehensive Guide. LD Wilson Consultants, Inc., 1993

nervousness. Potassium is critical for normal nutrient transport into the cell – deficiency can result in muscular weakness, depression and lethargy. Excess sodium is associated with hypertension, but adequate amounts are required for normal health. Even vitamin status can be indirectly assessed from HTMA.

HTMA can detect recent exposure (from the last couple of months) of toxic metals in your blood that ultimately end up in the hair tissues as well. The way I use the test is to take an initial baseline sample to see the levels of minerals and toxic metals that are actively circulating in the blood during the last couple of months – this is basically the time it takes to grow the inch-and-a-half of hair that is taken.

I then put my patients on a natural chelator which I researched and invented – it is a natural chelator that has undergone double-blind, placebo-controlled trials with 350 people and is called HMD™. A further HTMA is taken after 2 months to see how many metals have been mobilized from storage sites in the body – usually we find a percentage increase of metals in the second test.

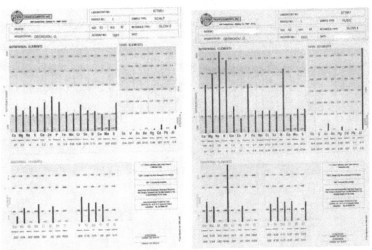

HTMA results two months apart after using HMD®

The two reports above are from the same patient, taken two months apart. On the left is the baseline sample before any natural chelator or minerals were given. Generally, there is a low level of minerals with a little Cadmium and Aluminium burden. This is what has been circulating in the blood over the last couple of months but is not a reflection of what is stored in the body tissues and organs. On the right are the results of the second hair test, taken two months after the first, while on the HMD™ protocol. Notice that there is a huge increase in the levels of aluminium with some arsenic also appearing – these are the heavy metals that were in the storage organs that were mobilized by the HMD™[20].

Preparing by Detoxifying

It is very important for the success of the Candida protocol that the internal milieu is balanced and clean. One of the quickest, cheapest and most efficient ways of achieving this is to undergo a 15-day alkaline detox programme using only fresh fruits, vegetables, vegetable juices and soups, steamed vegetables with olive oil and herbs, as well as herbal teas.

This is a summary table of the steps required to prepare for detoxifying. It is highly recommended that you take the supplements recommended as they are doctor-formulated and have been tried and tested in clinical practice by me personally. These are high quality and pure, but if you can find alternatives then this is fine.

We will discuss each of these supplements in more details below and examine their ingredients and their benefits.

---

[20] This protocol using a pre-post hair sample can be found at https://www.detoxmetals.com/use-hair-tests-clinical-decision-making/

STEPS IN DETOXIFICATION PROTOCOL

TASK	TIME TAKEN	Supplements needed	Comments
1. Alkaline Detoxificatio n	15 days	HMD MULTIS, KRILL OIL, HEPATO PLUS, VITAMIN C	www.worldwidehealthcenter.net
2. Parasite detox	15-30 days	PARAFORM PLUS ONE, BLACK WALNUT TINCTURE	www.worldwidehealthcenter.net
3. Liver/GB cleanse	1 day	MAGNESIUM MALATE, EPSOM SALTS	www.worldwidehealthcenter.net
4. Heavy Metal Detox	2 months	HMD™, LAVAGE, CHLORELLA	www.worldwidehealthcenter.net

There are toxins in the food you eat, the water you drink and the air you breathe. Even your own body produces toxins as a result of its many metabolic processes that keep you alive.

There are a number of benefits of detoxification:

•The digestive tract is cleansed of accumulated waste and fermenting bacteria.

•Liver, kidney and blood purification can take place, which is not possible during regular eating patterns.

•Mental clarity is enhanced as chemical and food additive overload is reduced.

•Reduced dependency on habit forming substances such as sugar, caffeine, nicotine, alcohol and drugs.

•The stomach size is returned to normal as bad eating habits can be stopped.

•The hormonal system is enhanced which is especially true for growth hormones.

• The immune system is stimulated.

After detoxifying on an alkaline diet for 15 days, patients report higher energy levels, clear and glowing skin, weight loss of several pounds, clear-headedness, reduced cellulite, good body tone and a great feeling of being relaxed.

Detoxification is the process of removing the toxins that have been accumulating in the body tissues and organs throughout a person's life. These toxins will have been acting as metabolism blockers by literally poisoning the cells and not allowing them to function correctly.

Before we look at the details, here is a summary table that will help you under the various steps that you need to follow.

Some of these supplements I give to all patients as part of a repair and rejuvenation process – these would include a high-potency multivitamin/mineral formula such as HMD MULTIS, KRILL PLUS, which is a good source of omega 3 fatty acids, but with a lower probability of being high in mercury.

I encounter almost 80% or more of my patient having digestive issues – bloating and distension in the stomach and the intestines, so I will give <u>DIGEST PLUS</u> which are pancreatic enzymes that will help gut digestion, and <u>BETAINE COMPLEX</u> which contains hydrochloric acid for digesting concentrated proteins in the stomach.

For those that are doing the liver and gallbladder cleanse, then <u>MAGNESIUM MALATE</u> is important in order to soften the stones before the cleanse as drinking apple juice which contains malic acid is too sweet and will feed the Candida.

TYPICAL DETOXIFICATION & REJUVENTATION SUPPLEMENT SHEET

REMEDY	MORNING	LUNCH	DINNER	COMMENTS
HMD MULTIS Multivitamin mineral	2	2	0	With food
KRILL OIL Fatty acids – omega 3	1	0	1	With food
DIGESTIZYME Pancreatic enzymes – gut digestion	1	1	1	With main meals only
GASTRIC AID Hydrochloric acid – stomach digestion	1	1	1	With main meals only
HEPATO PLUS Liver detox herbal formula	1	1	1	With food 15 – 30 days only
PARAFORM PLUS ONE Parasite detox herbal formula	1	1	1	Away from food
MAGNESIUM MALATE Softens gallbladder stones	1	1	1	With food, for 15 days only
HMD Heavy metal detox chelator	45 drops	45 drops	45 drops	In a little water or juice
LAVAGE Herbal drainage remedy	25 drops	25 drops	25 drops	Away from food
LUGOL'S IODINE Feeds the thyroid	2 drops	0	2 drops	
WALNUT TINCTURE Parasite detox herbal formula	2 tsp	0	0	
CHLORELLA Clears toxic metals from matrix and gut	2	0	2	With food
Alpha Lipoic acid Water & Fat soluble antioxidant	1	0	1	With food
IF CONSTIPATED:				
CONSFORM Herbal formula for constipation	1	1	1	With food

CHAPTER 5:

The Da Vinci Centre

Detoxification Diet

We suggest that the person eat only fresh fruit, salads, freshly squeezed juices, steamed vegetables and vegetable soups for 15 consecutive days.

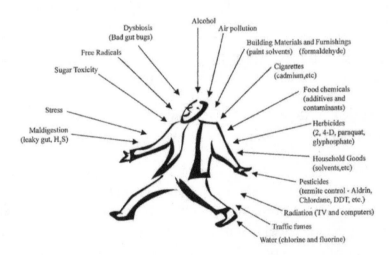

These are the foods that are allowed during the detoxification phase, no other family of foods is allowed. You may eat as many of the following foods as you wish, but it is best to eat only when you feel hungry. Wash all fruit and vegetables in a bowl of water with 4-5 tablespoons of grape vinegar added to help wash away any pesticide/ herbicide residues. Rinse afterwards with clean water. Here are the foods that you can eat in plenty:

1.Salads – use any type of fresh vegetables you like, in any combination. Use organic vegetables when available and include bean sprouts when in season. Salad dressings should be kept simple - a little virgin olive oil with fresh lemon, or cider vinegar. Add plenty of fresh onion and garlic - these are very detoxifying.

2.Steamed vegetables – eat any variety you like, including broccoli, cauliflower, potatoes, beetroot, carrots etc. Steam as opposed to boil, and eat with a little herbal salt, lemon and a little virgin olive oil, with plenty of garlic.

3.Vegetable soups - of all kinds, but broccoli, leak and vegetable soups are fine.

4.Stir-Fried Vegetables – again, any type of vegetables are fine, cooked in their own juices using a Wok.

5.Vegetable juices - drink a minimum of 1-3 per day and try to include one cocktail comprising one-third of a glass of raw green juice (spinach, parsley, cabbage and any other green vegetables), with a small beetroot, topped up with carrot juice. Carrot juice has a strong effect on the digestive system, provides energy, serves as an important source of minerals, promotes normal elimination, has diuretic properties and helps to build healthy tissue, skin and teeth.

6.Fresh Fruit - choose the fruit of your choice and eat as much as you like, whenever you like. You could begin the day with 2-3 pieces of fruit, which are gentle on the digestive system. Make a tasty fruit salad.

Try to avoid too many juicy fruits as this may overly feed the Candida, and certainly avoid all forms of fruit juices as this will give sugar to the body quickly, again feeding the Candida. Avocados provides a good source of protein. There is tremendous benefit in adding fruit during the detox due to their living enzymes and phytonutrients which are very cleansing to the body. Remember, we are not treating the Candida yet, only helping the body to cleanse and prepare for the 3-month Candida protocol.

7.Fresh Nuts – it is generally OK to have some fresh nuts such as almonds and walnuts.

8.Herbal teas - any of your choice. Chamomile is a good relaxant; aniseed and mint are good for the digestive system; Kombucha, dandelion tea is excellent for purifying the blood and detoxifying and stimulating liver function; sage tea is a blood cleanser; nettle tea is excellent for driving away excess fluid out of the tissues and is a wonderful cleanser for all the detoxification organs. Drink as many as you like, with a little honey on the tip of a teaspoon if you like.

The purpose of this diet is to detoxify – to remove the toxins from the fat cells and tissues as well as the organs, so that the body can return to its optimum level of functionality.

You will also need to drink at least 8-10 glasses per day of still mineral water to flush out the toxins – this is VERY IMPORTANT, so please take note!

When the 15 days are over, you should carry on eating the above for a couple more days while gently adding a little protein such as fresh steamed or grilled fish, organic chicken, pulses, a soft-boiled organic egg or a little cheese. Go gently on the protein for a couple of days before you begin eating normally again so that you do not overload your digestive system.

Parasites, Heavy Metals and Other Toxins

As part of the detoxification process, the Da Vinci Center also attempts to detoxify heavy metals that can easily be detected using a hair analysis, as already mentioned above.

One of the most researched natural chelators in the world that has undergone double-blind, placebo-controlled trials with 350 people is called HMD™. It has been shown to safely chelate many different types of heavy metals, including uranium, a difficult metal to chelate. It was invented by me and there are a number of scientific papers written in peer-reviewed journals – Scientific Research on Natural Heavy Metal Chelators: Testing What Works and Natural Heavy Metal Chelators: Do They Work?[1]

Dr. Hulda Clark, Ph.D., N.D., a naturopathic physician, has brought the issue of parasitically-caused diseases and other types of toxicity back into the spotlight in recent years, dealing with this subject at length in her book: "The cure for all diseases". Dr. Hulda describes various methodologies and procedures to cleanse the body from these nasty creatures. Check out this questionnaire (in Appendix) to see whether you are likely to have a parasite load.

The Herbal Parasitic Cleanse

There are some good herbal formulas that are designed to eradicate parasites.

One such formula that I use and formulated is called PARAFORM PLUS ONE (one capsule, three times daily, away from food). It contains a number of powerful anti-parasitic herbs that are suitable for vegetarians, such as:

Magnesium caprylate

---

[1] https://www.detoxmetals.com/research/

Cinnamon powder

Cloves powder

Shiitake mushroom powder

Garlic powder extract (10000mg/g)

Glucomannan (95%)

Pumpkin seed P E 4:1 (40%) (equivalent to 200mg pumpkin seed powder)

Chicory root P.E 4:1 (equivalent to 120mg chicory root powder)

Grapefruit seed P.E 5:1 (equivalent to 100mg grapefruit seed powder)

Cayenne extract 7:1 (equivalent to 100mg cayenne powder)

Fenugreek seed P.E 4:1 (equivalent to 48mg fenugreek seed powder)

Olive leaf extract 15:1, 6% Oleurpein (equivalent to 50mg olive leaf powder)

It is a powerful formula that we have been using with good results in clinical practice, and goes well when combined with **PARAFORM TINCTURE**, another powerful anti-parasitic herb – 2 teaspoons in the morning in a little water, away from food.

Bioresonance Devices

As well as using herbal formulas to eradicate parasites, I recently have added other protocols using Bioresonance devices, researched by Russian scientists who developed a powerful, portable, programmable Bioresonance device called the DEVITA MINI AP – this has undergone considerable trials from the Russians who purport its success in eradicating a number of parasites and microorganisms.

I have been using Bioresonance devices for many years now, but the innovation of the Russian devices is that they are portable, no larger than a mobile phone, and can be programmed to resonate with individual parasites and other microorganisms. There is also the DEVITA MINI RITM that is for upregulating the organ systems.

If we take a crystal wine glass as an example, this has its own resonant frequency, of around 500 Hertz. If we can produce a sound at the same frequency and stand the glass in front of a speaker, then the glass will absorb this frequency and break. This is the phenomenon of RESONANCE.

In the same way, microbes also have their own resonant frequencies – if we can match these frequencies then the microbes will absorb this energy and burst. You can see this happening in the video below with frequencies killing a parasite.

Treatment with the devices is based on the principles of Bioresonance. They are as close as we can get to the Hippocratic Oath that says: "Do no harm" when treating people. These gentle devices achieve exactly this – they can heal without being invasive and causing side-effects.

Checkout a presentation at an international conference on YouTube talking about "Alternatives to Antibiotics"

https://youtu.be/bYcvs4blUq8

The devices also have the approval of the Ministry of Health of Russia, as well as Israel and Germany where they are presently manufactured with CE approval as wellness devices. These devices also have patents in 73 different countries as well as more than 117 scientific research studies backing it in the last 20 years – see www.deta-elis-uk.com

The Secrets to Success

It is my opinion, if one wants to be successful at eradicating Candida, that you must eradicate the pathogen using natural anti-fungal remedies, while at the same time cleaning up the internal milieu.

One further key to success is the important step of converting the pathogenic, mycelial Candida back to the normal budding yeasts – this is a **crucially important step** often missed by many practitioners of natural medicine. The only remedies that can do this successfully are the Sanum isopathic fungal remedies that have been invented by Professor Enderlein after many years of experimentation using darkfield microscopy.

Many physicians now believe that an interim measure before embarking on any treatment should be a protocol for Candida overgrowth; this possesses such a minor risk and expense that it should be considered in any chronic illness.

One clinical trial a person may try is to avoid certain foods for five days that are known to facilitate the growth of yeast. Such foods include the following:

•**SUGAR and SIMPLE CARBOHYDRATES** such as those found in all sweetened food including honey, molasses, sorghum, maple syrup, sugar, fructose, maltose, dextrose, corn syrup, etc.

•**YEAST PRODUCTS** such as beer, wine, yeast leavened bread, natural B vitamins, brewer's yeast

•**FERMENTED and MOULDY FOODS** such as mushrooms, cheese, vinegar, mustard, catsup, relish and other condiments made with vinegar.

After avoiding these foods for 5 days, try adding them back into the diet in large quantities. By observing how one feels while off these foods, in comparison to any adverse effects experienced when going back on the foods, one may get a clue as to any possible yeast involvement as a causative factor for any adverse symptoms.

If adverse symptoms are provoked by a return to the yeast enhancing foods, your physician may feel that there is at least a possible reason to suspect Candida overgrowth, which may then warrant more definitive action.

This may not be the best method and personally I do not use it as I will use VRT Bioresonance screening and ART to determine whether there is pathogenic Candidiasis, backed up by the signs and symptoms using Dr. Crook's Candida Questionnaire. However, if you are not a Bioresonance practitioner or use any other form of ANS testing, then this may be a good way to begin.

Detoxification Symptoms – "The Healing Crisis"

When the body detoxifies it goes through various biochemical and physiological changes[21]. Generally, on the first day of fasting, the blood sugar level is likely to drop below 65-70 mg/dl. The liver immediately compensates by converting glycogen to glucose and releasing it into the blood. After a few hours, the basal metabolic rate is likely to fall in order to conserve energy. This means that the heart, pulse and blood pressure will drop. More glycogen may be used from muscles, causing some weakness.

As the body requires more energy, some fat and fatty acids are broken down to release glycerol from the glyceride molecules and are converted to glucose. You may notice the skin becoming quite oily as these fatty acids and glycerol increase in the blood. The skin is one of the largest detoxification organs, so you may get some skin problems such as pimples, acnes or a pussy boil – this is all part of the body trying to cleanse. The complexion may become pallid for a day or two as the wastes accumulate in the blood. The incomplete oxidation of fats may result in the formation of Ketones, resulting in ketoacidosis. Combined with high levels of urea resulting from protein metabolism, this state can cause a number of symptoms which may suppress appetite, as they affect the satiety centre in the hypothalamus. Generally, this takes a few days to happen and you may notice your appetite dwindling. You may get pains in different joints, or organs such as the lungs. There may be a considerable amount of yellow mucus released from the throat and expelled. The sinuses may also begin clearing with more mucus secreted.

Given that the body is releasing these toxins quickly during the first few days of the detoxification process, it should not surprise us to experience some changes in our bodies that may cause certain symptoms. Initially, for the first 2-3 days, these symptoms can be a little unpleasant, SO BE WARNED! A fair number of people will have headaches, nervousness, diarrhea, upset stomach, energy loss, furry tongue, halitosis (bad breath), as well as acne or other skin rashes, a general feeling of malaise, frequent urination due to the toxins irritating the bladder, and some of their existing symptoms may be exacerbated. When the toxic residues enter the blood, they affect mind and body functions.

These may be unpleasant symptoms for the first couple of days, but they are a NORMAL part of the detoxification process, and in natural medicine we call this the HEALING CRISIS or HERXHEIMER REACTION. All these symptoms indicate that the DETOX IS WORKING! This is a temporary and transient crisis, it will pass – so hang on in there and don't worry that there is something wrong with you, apart from the fact that you are loaded with toxins.

There was always something wrong with you, and now you are doing something about it – you are reversing this toxic process that your body has adapted to, but that is not healthy. If you are a coffee drinker, then the symptoms will be more pronounced, as your body will be in a state of withdrawal. Yes, coffee is a drug, and when you come off it you go into withdrawal, meaning that your body will start asking for a dose of what it is addicted to. When it doesn't get it, then it screams for it louder and louder, usually in the form of headaches, migraines, muscle pains, general weakness and lack of concentration.

Enduring a cleansing crisis is the hardest part of the healing process. To stop feeling bad, most people want to eat - but do not eat during a cleansing crisis. The body is overloaded with the work of removing toxins. Digestion makes matters worse. Drinking one or two glasses of sodium bicarbonate (baking soda) – one teaspoon in each glass drunk twice daily - will help to neutralize the ketoacidosis.

Helter-Skelter rides are common – the 'downward slope' is when the body is vigorously cleansing, and the blood gets swamped with toxins causing you to feel down, moody, depressed, achy – like having a bad cold. You feel weak and lethargic. The mind rationalizes: 'I feel horrible: this can't be working.' You can maintain a normal routine of work on a dip, but it requires willpower and determination. It also helps to know that the longer the down period, the greater the fasting high.

Phases of Detoxification

There is a lot going on in the body during the detoxification process – most of the work is happening in the largest detoxification organ of the body – the liver. The detoxification phases in the liver are composed of two phases known as Phase I and Phase II. These phases chemically bio-transform toxins into progressively more water-soluble substances through a series of chemical reactions so that they can be excreted from the body.

Supplements That Help the Detoxification Pathways

Some of the nutrients required for the proper functioning of the detoxification pathways have already been mentioned above. To reiterate, it is strongly advised that you drink at least 10 large glasses of mineral or reverse osmosis water daily (about 2 litres), so that you can flush out the toxins quicker. It is also wise to take a multivitamin formula such as the HMD MULTIS that we have formulated and have tested clinically, to help optimize your levels of vitamins and minerals, which are crucial raw materials for many of the detoxification pathways of the body. Make certain that you choose one that has high levels of vitamins and minerals, not just the RDA levels.

Taking between 1-2 grams of Vitamin C daily during the detoxification process will also help to absorb certain toxins, as well as helping the immune system cope with a heavy burden of toxins that it needs to get rid of. I usually recommend a Calcium/Magnesium Ascorbate VITAMIN C BLEND caps, which is an alkaline form of vitamin C, and is much gentler on the stomach and gut than plain ascorbic acid. These ones are in capsule form as many people prefer capsules than powder, but you can always open the capsules and pour their powder into some juice – two of these are equivalent to about 2 grams.

There are also herbs that you can take that can help upregulate the detoxification pathways of the liver and the kidneys, such as one that we formulated and works well in clinical practice called HEPATO PLUS . Take one capsule three times daily with food; the ingredients per capsule are:

Per capsule:

Artichoke extract (40:1), 2.5% cynarin (equivalent to 4800mg of fresh artichoke)
Parsley powder
Beetroot extract (5:1) (equivalent to 400mg of fresh beetroot powder)
Turmeric powder (95% Curcumin)
Burdock root extract (5:1) (equivalent to 200mg of fresh burdock root)
Fennel seed extract (4:1) (equivalent to 120mg of fresh fennel seed powder)
Dandelion root extract (4:1) (equivalent to 100mg of fresh dandelion root powder)
Liquorice root extract (5:1) (equivalent to 100mg of fresh liquorice)

N-acetyl L-cysteine

Alpha lipoic acid

Garlic (black aged garlic) extract (100:1) (equivalent to 500mg of fresh garlic powder)

Ginger root powder

Cayenne (Capicum Frutescens) extract (8:1) (equivalent to 30mg of fresh cayenne powder)

The concentrated active herbal ingredients in this comprehensive food based formula help to cleanse a congested liver and gallbladder and support cell repair and protection.

Formulated to stimulate, flush, cleanse and protect these two important organs. If you thought milk thistle worked well, this formula will "blitz" internal congestion and toxins.

Where there is a history of constipation, we also use a herbal formula called COLFORM..

COLFORM is a well-known herbal colon cleanser and bowel support combination, based on a formula by master herbalist, Dr. John R. Christopher.

Popular with colonic hydrotherapists, COLFORM contains a range of active herbal ingredients which help to cleanse the intestinal tract, soften the stool, stimulate the liver and improve peristalsis. This, in turn, helps to produce bowel movements and expel layers of old encrusted mucus and faecal matter that may have accumulated over time.

It acts to gently cleanse, stimulate and tone the bowel wall, supporting a move towards unassisted bowel movements.

In similar cases, we use another formula that is also very good at helping to balance dysbiosis called OXYGUT .

OXYGUT is a powerful, yet gentle, non-habit-forming colonics formula, with nutrients specifically selected to contribute to an increase in faecal bulk and normal bowel function.

It contains: magnesium peroxide, magnesium oxide, magnesium hydroxide, sugar beet fibre, ascorbic acid (Vitamin C), citric acid, citrus bioflavonoids, apple cider vinegar powder (a natural digestive) and fructo-oligosaccharides (FOS, a prebiotic) – ingredients designed to support the 'oxygenating' actions of the magnesium, as well as digestive regularity. It is a natural approach to supporting long-term bowel health and ideal as part of a cleanse and detox programme – take 2 capsules on an empty stomach, once to twice per day, but you can try increasing these to 3 capsules twice daily if this is a comfortable dosage for you.

Another product that we use that is a herbal tincture, that is designed as a drainage remedy is called HMD™ LAVAGE.

It is one thing MOBILIZING toxins from the body, it is another ELIMINATING them – this requires efficient detoxification organs, and therefore DRAINAGE REMEDIES are as important as detoxification remedies that mobilize toxins, but do not necessarily facilitate their removal.

This herbal drainage remedy has been specifically formulated to open up your detoxification organs and support your kidneys and liver during detox. It will help your body eliminate metals and toxins faster and more efficiently. HMD™ LAVAGE is anti-bacterial and anti-inflammatory as well as a powerful antioxidant specifically developed for ultimate detoxification. Dosage for adults: 25 drops 3x per day, in a little water, away from food.

Stay with the Detoxification Process

Stay with the detoxification process, and allow yourself time to rest, particularly during the first few days. Therefore it is best starting on a

Friday, given that you will have the weekend at home to get organized and rest when you need to.

Vigorous exercise during this initial period may be difficult due to tiredness created from the toxins themselves, so there is no need to push yourself. Perhaps a 20-30-minute walk with a friend or loved one in an open-air park is fine. You need to conserve your energy levels for the detoxification process. Under normal circumstances, the body uses 80% of its energy for detoxification, which is a substantial amount, and this will increase during the 15 days of this intensive detox programme. Having said this, many people who have efficient detoxification organs that are not so congested can often do more vigorous exercise and they feel great for it. Exercise is certainly to be encouraged, but there is no need to push yourself during the detoxification process if your body is telling you otherwise.

The Good News

The good news is that after the initial healing crisis you WILL FEEL A LOT BETTER. This is literally a guarantee that I can give you personally, as I have witnessed this hundreds of times with my patients, as well as myself. I personally detoxify twice a year for 15 days, and another 7 days in the summer when fruit and juices are plentiful here in Cyprus.

I KNOW how it feels when your body begins to get rid of the toxins and you are over the healing crisis – a clarity of mind that is crystal clear, increased concentration, increased energy levels, better sleep, calmer, more reflective state of being, increased awareness of your environment, better digestion, your constipation improves, body pains dwindle or melt away, arthritis improves, chests and throats clear, skin colour and tone greatly improves and I have had many clients who cut down or actually stopped smoking, as the body rebels harder during a detox programme

These are all benefits that you will experience, so STICK WITH THE PROGRAMME and achieve OPTIMUM HEALTH. Once you experience this state of optimum health you will wonder what the hell you were doing when you had moderate health, just like most people walking the planet today. The Alkaline Detox Diet is one of the most positive steps you can take and should be treated and enjoyed that way – treat yourself for 15 days, eat as much as you like, whenever you like, of the foods that you are allowed during the detox.

<u>Before</u> Starting the Detox Programme

There are a few indications which would exclude some people from starting the detox programme and they should not do so if any of the following apply:

• You are pregnant – the toxins released during the detoxification process can harm the embryo, as the embryo's capacity to detoxify is limited due to its poor organ functionality at such early stages of development.

• You are breastfeeding – toxins released into the mother's blood will travel to the milk, so the baby will get a dose of toxic milk that will not help them in any way. Wait until after the baby is weaned off the breast and meanwhile you could start eating healthily.

• You are presently being treated for an illness or condition such as diabetes or heart problems without medical supervision. It is important for your doctor or health practitioner to know what you are doing. With diabetics, for example, it is possible that you might go into a hypoglycemic episode where your blood sugar levels fall below normal, due to the increased insulin production by the pancreas. I have seen this several times – as the pancreas begins to clear of toxic overloads, it begins to function better, so it can begin to produce MORE insulin than before, resulting in a sudden decrease of blood sugar levels. This is fine as long as a health practitioner is aware of what is going on, and can adjust the dosage of drugs to suit.

• You are recovering from a serious illness without expert medical supervision – if you are recovering from cancer, any type of operation, an accident or other serious disease, then you should be extremely careful of detoxifying by yourself, as the toxins released in the body could upset the healing process and period of convalescence. Seek guidance from an experienced health practitioner who has experience in detoxifying. It is pointless asking a doctor who has no idea of detoxifying, as you are more than likely going to get a negative report, just from pure ignorance. Seek the help of an experienced person in these matters and take note that not many medical doctors are knowledgeable of the detoxification process, nor have experience in these matters. Only very few do, so do not take it for granted that all are knowledgeable because they are doctors.

• You are taking any prescribed or non-prescribed medication – again, the toxins mixed with the drugs could exacerbate further the healing crisis and cause more symptoms than are necessary.

• You are not ready at this moment in time to begin – the detox programme does require a little discipline and organization so would not be suited to a person who is travelling continuously, or eating out continuously with business associates, or who is under a particular stress from marital or domestic problems. We need to prepare ourselves psychologically and emotionally as well before we begin. If you feel that this is not the right time for you, then postpone it for another time when you are.

Preparing for the Detox

Preparing for the detox is not difficult, nor is it costly, but should be done some time BEFORE you decide to begin. There are a number of things that you need to gather before you start. A checklist of essentials is outlined below:

• A large stock of fresh vegetables and fruit in season – kept in the fridge for freshness. If you have access to ORGANIC FRUIT and

VEGETABLES, then this should be your obvious first choice. Organic produce is free from the pesticides and chemical fertilizers that are harmful to the body but are also richer in nutrients due to the organic fertilizers that are used. One famous doctor, Dr. Gerson, said that 'The soil is our second metabolism.' What he meant by this profound statement was that the nutrient quantity and quality of the soil is going to determine the quality of our bodily functioning or metabolism. Organic produce has been 'fed' the right ingredients of minerals, trace elements and vitamins that our bodies require to function optimally. I sincerely wish I had a steady supply of organic produce at my disposal here in Cyprus where I work and live, but unfortunately, we are not that health conscious as a nation to begin organic farming as of yet.

• A good thermos flask – you can use this for transporting freshly squeezed fruit or vegetable juices to and from work. It is important to remember, however, that the live enzymes and vital energy in freshly squeezed juices has a life-span of ONLY THREE HOURS. So, it is crucial that you drink the juice within these 3 hours and try to keep the juice as cool as possible – heat can destroy these very vulnerable enzymes. You may also use the flask to transport herbal teas, either hot or cold (with ice cubes) if you wish.

• A good quality juicer – there are many different types of juicers on the market, and it is a true science to choose the right one. Most of the juicers on the market for domestic use are centrifugal juicers. If you are buying one try to find the best that money will buy as this is going to be a sound health investment that will see you through many years of life. There are cheaper ones at half the price that will probably only last a year or less, so choose carefully. You could pick up a good one for less than $100, but if you can pay to buy the Rolls Royce of juicers, go for something like a Champion juicer (about $300), which will extract 25% more nutrients from vegetables and juices than the centrifugal juicer. The Champion juicer is a masticating juicer – it grinds the fruit or vegetable into a paste before spinning at high speed, to squeeze the juice through a screen set into the juicer bottom. The ultimate in juicers is the Health Stream Press which can extract up to 50% more juice than a centrifugal juicer but can cost from $500 to over $2,000 for the automated press.

• A steamer – metal (stainless steel) or bamboo – the type you place over or in the pan of hot water to steam vegetables. Steaming is far preferable to boiling as when you boil vegetables in water, they lose minerals such as potassium, which is crucial to health. Steaming vegetables decreases the losses of these important minerals.

• Olive oil – use extra virgin olive oil – this is extracted using a cold press method from whole, ripe, undamaged olives. It is made without heat and is unrefined, as compared with olive oil that is not virgin or extra virgin. It still contains many of the natural factors unique to olives, which are normally lost through degumming, refining, bleaching and deodorizing. Virgin olive oils do not suffer nutrient losses and molecular changes that negatively affect human health. Choose this oil over ones that do not have the word 'virgin' or 'extra virgin' on the label.

• Fresh garlic – have plenty of fresh garlic at hand - it would be wise to eat one clove a day as this contains more than 200 chemical compounds, most of them having therapeutic qualities. Eating fresh parsley and lemon juice or sucking on a whole clove can help to neutralize garlic odor on the breath. Garlic can inhibit and kill bacteria, fungi and parasites; lower blood pressure, blood cholesterol and blood sugar; prevent blood clotting, protect the liver and contains anti-tumor properties. It can also boost the immune system to fight off potential disease and maintain health.

Regarding detoxification, which particularly interests us here, garlic can stimulate the lymphatic system, which expedites the removal of waste from the body. In the meantime, it can nourish most of the organs such as the heart, stomach, circulation and lungs, as well as protect the cells from damage by nasty free radicals (molecules that harm the body). The Sulphur elements in garlic also help to stimulate certain enzyme systems that are beneficial for detoxifying such as the liver's glutathione pathways, which help to remove toxins from the body - there are going to be plenty of these passing through the liver in the next 15 days. So, now you understand why garlic is so important – it is one of the true wonders of nature, and I cannot understand why people dismiss it because of its odor, yet we accept so many other disgusting smells such as smokers smelling like ashtrays!

• A brush made of natural fibre – this is going to be used for SKIN BRUSHING (see details below).

• Water – you will need a large supply of either mineral or distilled water throughout the detoxification process. I suggest that you drink at least 10 glasses daily – this may mean having a glass next to you at home and the workplace and keeping it topped up. You will be surprised how many glasses you can drink in a day if you do this systematically. It really is a matter of habit, but what I have found is that if you don't have the water to hand, you will not remember to drink. Water is crucial to detoxification, as it is part of the flushing process, in order to get the toxins that are released by the cells out of the body. After a lot of research regarding water filters, I have personally settled for the reverse osmosis unit with a vortex energizer in circuit to put the proper right-spin quality back – there are many companies now that can fit the unit under your sink and add a separate small tap specifically for the drinking water. This is connected to your tap water, but the reverse osmosis filter will eliminate literally everything from chlorine, fluoride, heavy metals, pesticide residues as well as micro-organisms – it is squeaky clean water that you can drink and cook with – more on this later below.

• Fresh lemons or cider vinegar – what you use is really a matter of taste, but both are excellent and healthy condiments. Cider vinegar made from apples is very rich in potassium, a mineral that is required by all cells during metabolism. In his book, 'Cider Vinegar' by Cyril

Scott, he talks about how cider vinegar can help overweight people, citing several case histories. He recommends two teaspoons of cider vinegar in a tumbler of water, to be taken on rising in the morning. Exactly how it works is an enigma, but even if it does not work for weight loss, it will certainly help to alkalize the blood, which is normally acidic in most people, and will help to clean it.

• Herbal teas – there are a number of herbal teas that you could drink every day throughout the detox programme. Green tea is excellent, and apart from being rich in vitamin A, E, C, calcium and iron, it contains healthy phytonutrients called Epigallocatechin Gallate (EGCG), which inhibits the growth of cancer and lowers cholesterol levels. Dandelion 'coffee' is also excellent, as this herb purifies the blood, detoxifies and stimulates the function of the liver and is a natural diuretic. It is good to drink teas that help to drain the detoxification organs and get rid of the toxins. Another good one is stinging nettle tea, which helps to drive away excess fluid out of the tissues and helps with metabolism by increasing the elimination through the kidneys. Other goodies are chamomile, peppermint, rosehip, blackcurrant, elder flower, strawberry and Melissa. Most of these can be found in good health food shops – either in tea bags, or loose.

Major Detoxification Centres of the Body

The toxins will be released through four major detoxification centres of the body – the more you can help these detoxification pathways to open up, the less detox symptoms you will have. The major detoxification organs/centres of the body are:

1. Skin – excretes toxins such as DDT, heavy metals and lead through sweat. Skin brushing and saunas, as well as infrared saunas, are good ways of opening up the skin pores in order for toxins to be released.

2. Liver – filters the blood to rid it of bacteria; secretes bile to rid the blood of cholesterol, hemoglobin breakdown products and excess calcium. It also gets rid of prescription drugs from amphetamines,

digitalis, nicotine, sulphonamides, acetaminophens, morphine and diazepam. There are good herbs that can open up the detox channels in the liver such as dandelion (Taraxacum officinale), milk thistle (Silybum marianum), Green tea (Camellia sinensis), Artichoke (Cynara scolymus), Methionine, N-Acetyl Cysteine and Alpha lipoic acid and others. The herbal formula already mentioned has most of these and is called HEPATO PLUS .

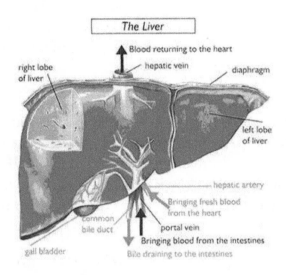

Food Enzymes and Detoxification

In order to remove the sludge and harmful waste from the body cells and tissues, it is important that you eat foods rich in live enzymes such as fresh fruits and vegetables and their fresh juices. These are dynamic catalytic substances that have the power to break down the fatty wastes stubbornly clinging to your fat cells and wash them out of the body. Food enzymes scrub your cells clean and therefore slim them down, and consequently slimming you down too.

Thorough chewing is a unique way of detoxifying the sludge from the mucous membranes of the gastrointestinal tract (GI). Whenever we chew, an enzyme called urogastrone is released which can help digest sludge present on the mucous membranes as well as offering a protective coating of the GI to protect against erosion.

Initially, scientists thought of enzymes as dead chemicals that merely acted as catalysts – making things work faster. Since then, the works of people like Dr. Edward Howell: 'Enzyme nutrition' and Anthony Cichoke: 'Enzymes and Enzyme Therapy,' has shown that enzymes are indeed very much alive and have lots of stored potential energy. As Dr. Howell states in his book, "They are protein carriers charged with vital energy factors, just as your car battery consists of metal plates charged with electrical energy."

These enzymes help you to digest your food, to absorb nutrients into your bloodstream and to dispatch nutrients to every part of your body. Without enzymes, there would be no life! These live enzymes with this vital energy come only from raw, live foods or their juices. Since good health depends on all metabolic enzymes doing an excellent job, we must make sure that nothing interferes with the body making enough of them.

One of the problems with maintaining the level of these enzymes is that they are very sensitive to heat – they are intolerant of heat. If water is hot enough to feel uncomfortable to the hand, it will injure enzymes in food. Nearly all of the food that we eat is cooked – most of it is cooked to death! Cooked food is deficient in enzymes with their vital energy. This means that you are also deficient in enzymes, which will lead to incompletely metabolized food (which is stored as waste in your adipocytes), giving you excess weight.

It is therefore crucially important to attack the stored-up sludge in your adipose tissue mass. So how do we get a good source of live enzymes? – we eat live, raw foods.

If there are digestive problems such as bowel distension, bloating, flatulence and wind, pain after eating – it would be wise to supplement a digestive enzyme with your food. You will find that as the food is digested your bloating will be a thing of the past in 15-20 days but carry on taking the digestive enzymes for at least 3 months.

If there are also a difficulty digesting protein concentrates such as meat and pulses, then this is an indication of hypochlorhydria or an insufficient production of hydrochloric acid by the stomach. This will cause stomach bloating, a feeling of heaviness after eating protein foods that will last many hours. This is because the stomach has to keep the food there for many hours in order to digest it correctly and you are likely to get fermentation, and wind will be expelled by the mouth. In this case, you will also need to take Betaine hydrochloric acid and Pepsin capsules with food.

The Theory of Autointoxication

The compelling suspicion that a stagnant bowel filled with putrefying matter can leak out and become a source of infection for the rest of the body, was first suggested by the ancient Egyptians. In the 19th century this became known as "The Theory of Autointoxication – self poisoning from one's own retained wastes." This idea has been enthusiastically embraced by every subsequent generation. One of the main causes is constipation.

Constipation

Constipation has done more to provide the health profession with an obvious solution to undiagnosable ailments than any other simple complaint. It is defined as 'The difficult or infrequent passage of feces' and it is associated with the presence of dry, hardened stools.

Constipation is a national pastime and slow bowels are more common today than years previous. For one thing, people not only ate better 100 years ago, they were more active and got outdoors more. When the bowels slow down, toxins are not eliminated but are reabsorbed and carried back to the liver for recycling and elimination. Reabsorbed bile salts have been linked to increased cholesterol levels – therefore, high cholesterol is a major precursor of constipation.

Also, when the bowels get slow and toxin levels increase, the pathogenic microorganisms grow to outnumber the normal flora, causing dysbiosis. Although friendly bowel flora such as Acidophilus (small intestine) and Bifidobacteria (colon) are needed to correct this, it is the clogged bowels that are the major problem. When the bowels move again, everything else will fall into order.

Our endocrine glands, which control metabolism, are also involved since it is our thyroid that controls metabolism, and metabolism affects how our bowels are functioning. In this way, constipation can be seen as a symptom of hypothyroidism. Low body temperatures (a symptom of hypothyroidism) are very common today –although they are not 'normal' – as many authors have reported.

Intestinal toxemia, which is a form of blood poisoning, is caused by the absorption of bacteria and their toxins through the intestinal wall.

The large intestine (colon) is the most prolific source of bacterial contamination in the entire body. Thirty-six toxic substances have been isolated from the human colon, including such compounds as indole, skatole, phenol and cresol. When these kinds of toxins are passing through the intestinal wall, they can enter the lymphatic or portal system and be directly transported to the liver. Temporary increases in the toxic load of the liver occur during periods of stagnation in the colon. Any prolongation of this state will impede the detoxification and bacteria killing function of the liver. The importance of this function cannot be overlooked when one realizes that blood from the intestinal tract enters the liver before it is delivered to the tissues of the body.

An overburdened liver, which cannot handle the toxic load from the intestine, transfers the task of detoxification onto another organ, the kidney. Unfortunately, the kidney is not able to reduce the amount and kind of toxins that enter the liver or to detoxify them as efficiently as the liver. The toxins that the kidneys do not remove from the blood, adversely affect the kidneys and increase circulating body-toxin levels.

The Oxford Dictionary defines constipation as 'Irregular and difficult defecation.' The question is, 'What is a regular bowel movement when there is no norm, and regularity becomes a meaningless expression when some people have a bowel movement regularly every Sunday morning, while others regularly empty their bowels after every meal?'

Defecation is a reflex action, stimulated by distension of the rectum with feces, but it is under voluntary control in adults and normally takes place only when time and circumstances are suitable. The presence of food in the stomach stimulates a reflex action called peristalsis, which moves food residue into and along the colon. Mass peristalsis gives us the feeling that we need to empty our bowels. This reflex action usually occurs after the first meal of the day but can also be stimulated by only drinking some liquid on rising.

If the call to defecate is persistently neglected, the reflex mechanism becomes less sensitive and constipation can result. This is likely to happen when there are time constraints causing hurry and stress (stress ceases peristaltic action in the colon). Also, when there are insufficient toilets or they are cold, dirty or inaccessible.

Some healthy people do not defecate every day and do not have any discomfort, and many others open their bowels every day with excruciating agony – passing dark, rock hard, compacted stools – and both cases would be considered constipated.

Ideally one should defecate as many times as we have a proper meal, usually 3 times per day, the main rule still being that we have a bowel movement at least once a day. The stool should be fibrous, light in colour, float in the water, break up easily and cause no pain or discomfort to pass – in fact no toilet paper should be needed. Pain or discomfort whilst passing hard or dry stool at less than daily intervals can be considered as constipation. Many people have suffered heart attacks as a result of vigorous efforts to have a bowel movement, as continuous efforts to evacuate material from the rectum increases the heart rate, blood pressure and respiration.

Referred to essentially as a Western disease, constipation is virtually unheard of among third world people adhering to traditional fibre-rich diets. Constipation is implicated in many Western diseases such as diverticulosis, obesity, varicose veins, cancer of the colon and rectum, appendicitis and hemorrhoids, all of which are very rare in the undeveloped countries.

Nature Needs Some Help and Urgently

In the U.S., approximately 80 million people suffer from bowel problems. 100-120,000 a year lose their lives – usually from bowel cancer. Colon cancer is the second leading killer in the Western World. Behind these statistics are also those saved by colostomies (surgical removal of the large intestine) – in the US only approximately 250,000 people a year. In UK and the rest of Europe, the numbers are more or less the same.

Bowel disorders, especially colon cancer, were unknown to our grandparents, and bowels experts all over the world now agree that poor bowel management is the root of most health problems. The faulty Western, commercialized diet is the focal point of the problem. A diet high in meat, white sugar, white flour, fat and low in dietary fibre and plain water (dehydration) is believed to be connected with constipation.

The root of the problem is clearly indicated by laxative sales, estimated at 600 – 800 million dollars a year. Statistics from the US and Europe are corresponding.

Laxatives aggravate the problem of constipation by interfering with the colon's ability to eliminate normally on its own. The chemicals within laxatives irritate and stimulate the colon to abnormally contract, in order to expel the irritating substances. In addition, the oral route of administration is the least optimal method for evacuation of the colon because crucial digestive processes occurring in the stomach and small intestine are interfered with. Most laxatives and purgatives precipitate dehydration. Hippocrates took the view of not disturbing and messing up the entire peptic system with harsh laxatives, as the problem lies at the extreme end of this same system. Standard enemas, even highly recommended as first aid, only cleanse the rectum and last portion of the colon, missing out most of the large intestine.

Colon Hydrotherapy is an extended and more complete form of an enema. This method extends beyond the rectum to cleanse the entire colon and offers greater therapeutic benefits. It addresses the cause or source of the constipation problem. Other methods treat only the symptoms and provide temporary relief of the problem.

The prevention of constipation may not seem of vital importance, except perhaps to the sufferer. However, there is substantial evidence to show that eating enough dietary fibre helps to prevent many bowel diseases as well as reducing the risk of heart disease, lowering cholesterol and blood pressure, improving blood sugar balance and maintaining a healthy gut flora.

Why constipated? – the biggest reasons? Dietary (lack of natural dietary fibre and consumption of devitalized foods, especially white sugar, white flour and all their by-products); neglecting the urge to eliminate; dehydration (too little water); stress; too little exercise (sitting for long hours); abuse of stimulants and drugs; irregular hours (work – rest, awake – asleep) and pathological conditions.

The most common signs and symptoms due to an impacted, constipated colon are:

☐ infrequent or difficult bowel movements; hard compacted stools and low stool weight;

☐ tiredness, fatigue, lethargy, lack of energy, poor concentration and irritability;

☐ bloating and flatulence; headaches, mental depression or dullness; Irritable Bowel Syndrome – IBS, diverticulosis, colitis, leaky gut, cancer of the bowel, Crohn's Disease, appendicitis, hiatus hernia; malabsorption – nutrient deficiency; bad breath and a coated tongue; hemorrhoids, varicose veins, obesity and cellulite.

Treating Constipation

Constipation should not be taken lightly! It is a huge burden on the entire body due to the high amounts of toxins leaking from the bowel into the blood stream, causing a huge toxic burden on the whole body.

We have already mentioned above certain herbal formulas that we use successfully to treat constipation and increase the transit time of the bowel to alleviate constipation. To reiterate, due to its importance, one powerful herbal formula is called CONSTFORM, the other is OXYGUT. The other herbal formula that can also be used if these two do not work is COLFORM.

I have never had a case of constipation that did not see benefit when 2 or all 3 of these remedies are combined – it is critically important to get the intestines mobile, emptying the toxic waste so that it is not constantly reabsorbed.

The first choice is the CONSTFORM which is a fast-acting colon cleanser, designed for the chronically constipated in need of strong treatment for a blocked bowel. Purgatives have been combined with carminatives to prevent griping.

It is a powerful intestinal cleanser, which will "blast loose" residual intestinal congestion and get any bowel cleanse program off to a good start.

The ingredients it contains are – can take up to 2 capsules x 3 times daily or adjust dosage to suit:

Rhubarb powder
Barberry powder
Glucomannan 90%
Alfalfa powder
Cayenne powder
Garlic powder
Aloe vera extract (200:1)
Dandelion root extract (4:1)
Ginger root extract (20:1)
Nettle leaf extract (4:1)

OXYGUT combines well with the CONSTFORM as it will help to eradicate many bad microbes that will be causing a dysbiosis, mainly due to the magnesium oxide "zapping" these microbes.

In addition, particularly for chronic cases of constipation, the COLFORM should also be added.

COLFORM contains a range of active herbal ingredients which help to cleanse the intestinal tract, soften the stool, stimulate the liver and improve peristalsis. This, in turn, helps to produce bowel movements and expel layers of old encrusted mucus and faecal matter that may have accumulated over time.

It acts to gently cleanse, stimulate and tone the bowel wall, supporting a move towards unassisted bowel movements.

Clearing Toxic Metals

Clearing toxic metals such as mercury from amalgams and fish, that will further aggravate the Candida, as well as cause free radical damage to many organs and tissues is also a wise step to take.

There are many products on the market that purport to detoxify heavy metals from the body, but none of them are supported by scientific research using correct methodologies known to scientific research. There is one natural product, however, that has been based on double blind, placebo-controlled research with over 350 people. It has also been used clinically by many practitioners around the world in the last 8 years or so. This is what I suggest can be used for most cases of heavy metal toxicity – I have called it the HMD ULTIMATE DETOX PACK and it consists of the following:

☐ HMD™ – 45 drops x 3 daily for adults[22] – sensitive adults who have chronic diseases or compensated detoxification organs, as well aspeople with neurological diseases such as multiple sclerosis and the like, as well as autistic people should begin with half this dose, or less, and increase by one drop x 3 daily, every day until they reach a comfortable level.

☐ HMD™ LAVAGE – this is a herbal formula of wild-crafted and organic herbs such as Silybum marianum (Milk Thistle Seed), Taraxacum officinale (Dandelion Root), Arctium lappa (Burdock Root), Trifolium pratense (Red Clover Tops), Curcuma longa (Turmeric Root), Hydrangea arborescens (Hydrangea Root) and Arctostaphylos uva ursi (Bearberry Leaf). This herbal formula is designed to facilitate detoxification of the liver, kidneys, lymphatics and skin, as well as cleanse the blood and act as a natural anti-inflammatory. Adult dosage: 25 drops x 3 daily for adults, or more as

---

[22] See www.detoxmetals.com/dosages for full details

directed by a practitioner.

☐ <u>HMD™ CHLORELLA</u> – there are many concerns about finding good quality, clean Chlorella that is void of heavy metals and xenobiotics. We have searched and travelled far and wide, and found an excellent source that is provided with a Certificates of Analysis with each pot. This chlorella comes from the western coast of Hai-Nan Island, China's southernmost island. Hai-Nan Island is a tropical island with an excellent climate and lies on the same latitude as Hawaii. The non-industrialized, pollution-free, tropical island offers favorable conditions for chlorella, including intense sunlight, pure water, and clean air. Available in 500mg tabs, adult dosage should be 2 tabs x 3 daily.

Chlorella is required in the gut to take it away toxic metals via the stools. If there is not enough chlorella, the neurotoxins are reabsorbed by the nerve endings in the gut wall and are at risk of being redirected to the spinal cord, and the brain.

Good quality chlorella lines the gut wall and mops up the free toxins found there. High toxicity and increasing symptoms need larger doses. This is very important and differs from the usual advice to reduce supplements if detoxing intensifies symptoms.

☐ <u>A-LIPOIC ACID</u> – I believe that when metals and other xenobiotics are mobilized in the body, there should be some protection against free radical damage. Lipoic acid is that extraordinary antioxidant which is both water and fat soluble, able to penetrate the brain and other nervous tissues, and is therefore able to protect all parts of the body against free radical damage.

I will often fine-tune this protocol depending on the needs of the patient, but generally this works well for most cases as a basic protocol.

Further Research

☐ During the 8 years of experience with HMD™ we have had many reports from women of all ages who have suffered from chronic endocrine problems, of coming back into balance while using HMD™ for 2-3 months. Many of these women suffered from irregular periods, heavy bleeding, PMS and other hormonal imbalances.

☐ Based on this anecdotal evidence we believe that HMD™ is eliminating other chemicals (xenobiotics) such as Bisphenyl A and Phthalates which are known endocrine-disrupting chemicals, as described above. Preliminary trials have already been done which have shown that indeed this is the case – HMD™ is eliminating the xenobiotics through the urine. However, the sample of people tested is small so further trials need to be conducted in this area before any scientific papers can be written.

CHAPTER 6:

The Da Vinci Candida Protocol (DCP)

Now that we have completed the preparation by detoxing on many different levels and preparing the internal milieu, we are now ready to begin examining in detail the Candida protocol in order to eradicate the Candida.

Even though I invented the protocol many years ago, it has come to be called the Da Vinci Candida Protocol as it has been implemented at the Da Vinci Holistic Health Center which I founded and run.

Let's take a conceptual look at the components of the Da Vinci Candida Protocol before we look at the details.

Please note, that we are aware that sourcing these products from different companies around the world is difficult and costly on freight charges. Rest assured, however, as you can purchase the complete package online from a one-stop shop www.worldwidehealthcenter.net.

The Da Vinci Candida Protocol has five basic objectives:

1.First, starve the Candida by eliminating the foods that feed it.

2.Second, kill the Candida using natural anti-Candida products that we will discuss below.

3.Repopulate the bowel flora with a high-potency Acidophilus and Bifidus probiotic that contains 60 billion live bacteria per capsule.

4.Regulate the dysbiosis and convert the pathological, mycelial form of Candida back to the normal form by the use of the SANUM remedies.

5.Restore biochemical balance to the body and strength to the immune system. This will allow the body once again to regain and maintain control over Candida growth by optimizing the diet – this would involve avoiding food intolerances and following the Metabolic Type Diet by Bill Wolcott. Also, eradicating parasites using herbal formulas that we discussed above as well as chelating heavy metals out of the system.

Here is a summary of the various steps that you need to follow to cure your Candida once and for all – even though it may be quite detailed, I can guarantee that if you follow it you will succeed, as have more than 5,000 patients that I have treated in the last 15 years or so. The success rate of eliminating the Candida approaches 100%, and by the time you have read all this book you will understand why.

STEPS IN CANDIDA PROTOCOL

TASK	TIME TAKEN	Supplements needed	Comments
1. Starve the Candida	3 calendar months		www.worldwidehealthcenter.net
2. Killing the Candida	3 calendar months	KANDIDAPLEX, HOROPITO, CAPRYLIC ACID, ACIDOPHILUS & BIFIDUS, CANDIDA 30C	www.worldwidehealthcenter.net
3. Repopulating friendly bacteria in gut	1 day	ACIDOPHILUS & BIFIDUS	www.worldwidehealthcenter.net
4. Using SANUM remedies to convert pathogenic Candida	2 months	SANUM REMEDIES	www.worldwidehealthcenter.net
5. Balancing body chemistry		VITAMIN C, GASTRIC AID, DIGESTIZYME,	www.worldwidehealthcenter.net

None of these objectives are mutually exclusive, nor can they be addressed in a serial way – they all need to be looked at concomitantly for the treatment protocol to be successful.

Let us now go through the various stages or phases of the Da Vinci Candida Protocol, beginning with a critically important stage – starving the Candida by not feeding it.

First Phase – Starving the Candida

I have found that it is literally impossible to treat Candida if one does not cut out **ALL** forms of sugar for a period of 3 months – this also includes natural fruit sugars or fructose. The foods that should be strictly **AVOIDED** for a 3-month period include:

1.SUGAR – and all foods that contain sugar. These include white and brown sugar, honey, syrups, liquors, lactose, fructose, all confectionary and sweet cakes, chocolates, ice-creams, home-made sweets and cakes, biscuits, fizzy beverages, all fruit drinks.

2.YEAST – all foods that contain yeast including breads, vinegar, ketchups, mayonnaise and pickles.

3.MUSHROOMS – all types, including Chinese mushrooms such as Shitake.

4.REFINED FOODS – all white flours, white rice, white pasta products, corn flour, custard and white cereal products, unless they are whole-meal or organic.

5.FERMENTED PRODUCTS – all alcoholic beverages, vinegar and all vinegar products such as ketchup, mayonnaise and pickles.

6.NUTS – all types of nuts that are cleaned and packaged without their shells – these have a tendency to collect fungal spores and molds from the atmosphere which will antagonize the Candida. Nuts that are fresh with their shells are OK.

7.FRESH AND DRIED FRUIT – all fresh fruit should be avoided for the initial **SIX WEEKS ONLY** as again, the fructose they contain will feed the Candida and make it extremely difficult to eliminate.

All other fruit that is not fresh such as cooked, tinned or dried and fruit juices should be avoided for the full 3 months – your health practitioner will advise you when to begin eating fruit again. Obviously, also avoiding fruit juices (vegetable juices are OK), as well as marmalades and dried fruits throughout the 3 months is important.

All other fruit that is not fresh such as cooked, tinned or dried and fruit juices should be avoided for the full 3 months – your health practitioner will advise you when to begin eating fruit again. Obviously, also avoiding fruit juices (vegetable juices are OK), as well as marmalades and dried fruits throughout the 3 months is important.

Second Phase – Killing the Candida

There are a number of herbal formulas, homeopathics and probiotics that are used in the Da Vinci Candida Protocol – they have been carefully selected after years of experimentation and the fact that they have worked time and time again with hundreds of people. The aim of using these supplements is to kill off the Candida - here is a table of these supplements in order, taken from one of the handouts that we give our patients, with an explanation on why and how they work later on.

REMEDY	MORNING	LUNCH	DINNER	COMMENTS
MAIN PROTOCOL				
CANDA PLUS	2	2	2	With meals
HOROPITO	1	0	1	With meals
ACIDOPHILUS & BIFIDUS	1	1	1	With meals
CANDIDA 30c	2pills	2pills	2pills	Dissolve in mouth Before meals
CAPRYLATE	1	1	1	With meals
Citricidal drops (Nail Fungus)	1 drop	0	1 drop	Under nails only
Natural Antibiotics				
NANO SILVER 50	1 tsp	1 tsp	1 tsp	Before food in water
OLIVE LEAF EXTRACT	1 tab	1 tab	1 tab	With meals
GRAPEFRUIT SEED EXTRACT	2 tabs	2 tabs	2 tabs	With meals
VITAMIN C BLEND	1-2 caps	1-2 caps	1-2 caps	With meals
TRIFORM	35 – 45 drops	35 - 45 drops	35 - 45 drops	Before food in water
PARAFORM PLUS TWO	1	1	1	With meals

R = Refrigerate

All the above-named products can be ordered from www.worldwidehealthcenter.net

* **The Natural Antibiotics** are only taken when there is an active infection such as a cold, flu or other infection. Take for 6 days **after** symptom withdrawal to make certain that all the bacteria have cleared from the body.

• **The Main Protocol** is taken for a full **3 months**.

•Two weeks after beginning the **Candida Protocol** the **SANUM remedies** must be begun.

Now let us look at the specific remedies in a little more detail to understand why and how they work to eradicate the Candida.

1.CANDA PLUS (was called **KANDIDAPLEX**) - a doctor-formulated compound that contains:

☐ Calcium undecylenate – 100 mg;

☐ Pau d'arco (Tabebuia avellanedae) bark extract 100 mg;

☐ Enlyse™ enzyme blend (cellulase, chitosinase, hemicellulase, protease, serrapeptase, amylase and lipase) 100 mg;

☐ Berberine (as berberine sulfate) 50 mg;

☐ Sorbic Acid 25 mg;

☐ Trans-Resveratrol (from Japanese knotweed (Polygonum cuspidatum) root extract) 10 mg.

Dosage 2 Capsules 3 x Daily

Each individual ingredient in CANDA PLUS has a specific function when it comes to eradicating Candida, as follows:

☐ Calcium undecylenate - undecenoic acid's ability to alter the composition of fatty acids in the cell membrane leading to an inability to sustain its fungal form.

☐ Pau D'Arco acts as a powerful antifungal agent. It contains several classes of compounds, lapachol, xyloidone and various napthaquinones. The most important of these is lapachol, which has been shown to inhibit the growth of Candida., that was similar to Amphotericin B.

☐ Enlyse™ – Enzymes such as Enlyse™ destroy the BIOFILM of Candida that we previously talked about, which is composed of protein polypeptides, polysaccharide carbohydrates, fibrinogen or fibrin and polynucleotides that contain RNA and DNA material. This structure is bound together with ligands that have stickiness properties.

☐ Berberine exhibits a broad spectrum of antibiotic activity. Berberine has shown antimicrobial activity against bacteria, protozoa, and fungi and upregulates immunity.

☐ Sorbic acid – inhibits fungi as well as molds – often found together in the body

☐ Trans-Resveratrol - exhibited antifungal activity against C. albicans and against 11 other Candida species. Also, inhibited the yeast-to-hyphae morphogenetic transition of C. albicans.

2. HOROPITO (practitioner-strength) – a New Zealand herbal product that contains two powerful anti-fungal agents that have been shown to kill Candida – Pseudowinterata colorata and the synergistic herb Aniseed that boosts effectiveness 6-fold. Dosage: 1 cap twice daily.

This natural herb, found mostly in New Zealand, has some amazing properties that have been scientifically researched.

Pseudowintera colorata, or mountain Horopito, is an evergreen shrub or small tree (1–2.5 m) commonly called pepperwood because its leaves have a hot taste.

Used by the indigenous Maori population of New Zealand - Infection due to Candida albicans is documented as once being a major cause of death of Maori babies, due to being fed an "unsatisfactory diet".

3.CAPRYLATE (500 mg) – a derivative of coconut that stops the Candida reproducing as well as killing the Candida. Dosage: 1-tab x 2 daily

4. CANDIDA 30c - homeopathic – helps to eradicate the Candida but using a different mechanism. Dosage: two pillules or one cap x 3 daily for 2 weeks only. These are stopped just as the Sanum remedies are begun.

Third Phase – Repopulating the Friendly Bacteria

This phase runs parallel with phase 2 and uses good quality, human strain probiotics such as the high-potency ACIDOPHILUS and BIFIDUS probiotics by Custom Probiotics, an American company. The Custom Probiotics formula that we use is a high count, multi strain Acidophilus and Bifidus probiotic dietary supplement containing 60 billion cfu's per capsule at the time of expiration. Resistant to stomach acids, with a slow die-off with temperature.

The Ingredients include 5 different strains of probiotics such as L. Acidophilus, L. Rhamnosus, L. Plantarum, B. Lactis, B. Bifidum.

There is considerable scientific evidence for activity of probiotics against a wide range of intestinal pathogens, including Candida species. Despite this, the mechanisms of effect have been poorly defined. However, it can be speculated that one or more of the following possible effects are in operation:

• competition for nutrients • secretion of antimicrobial substances (e.g. bacteriocins, peroxides) • reduction of gut pH • blocking of adhesion sites (Kennedy et al, 1985) • repression of virulence • blocking of toxin receptor sites • immune stimulation (local and systemic) • suppression of toxin production

To these supplements, we add a good-quality multivitamin such as HMD MULTIS to provide all the vitamins and minerals that the immune system requires for optimal functioning. Also, taking KRILL PLUS is helpful as this acts as a natural anti-inflammatory.

Phase 4 – Using SANUM-Isopathic Remedies to Normalize Pathogenic Candida

All of the above must be taken for the full 90 days of the protocol, with the exception of the Candida 30c. After two weeks of the anti-Candida diet, certain specialized isopathic remedies are introduced, known as SANUM remedies from Germany, after the work of the famous Prof. Enderlein. SANUM is a product system first developed in 1944 and is manufactured and distributed worldwide by the company SANUM-Kehlbeck in Germany.

SANUM therapy is widely recognized to positively influence the regulatory processes, the internal milieu, immune response capacity and the symbiotic bacterial ecology within the body. Each of these isopathic remedies are only taken a couple of times per week, with the exception of the Albicansan remedy that is taken day by day. The reason that we have spaced them out in the table below is that they tend to clash and antagonize each other, and cannot all be taken at the same time. So, if you follow the sequence in the table below, beginning from the specific day that you begin taking them, whether this is Monday, or Tuesday or Wednesday and so forth.

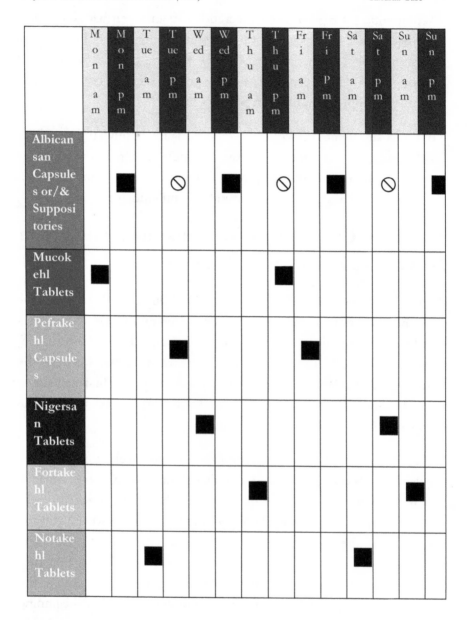

	M o n a m	M o n p m	T ue a m	T ue p m	W ed a m	W ed p m	T h u a m	T h u p m	Fr i a m	Fr i P m	Sa t a m	Sa t p m	Su n a m	Su n P m
Albican san Capsules or/& Suppositories		⬛		⊘		⬛		⊘		⬛		⊘		⬛
Mucokehl Tablets	⬛							⬛						
Pefrakehl Capsules				⬛				⬛						
Nigersan Tablets						⬛						⬛		
Fortakehl Tablets							⬛						⬛	
Notakehl Tablets			⬛								⬛			

Specifically, each of the 6 remedies is taken as follows:

☐ Albicansan ® (Candida albicans) – caps 4X - **1 cap every second day**.

☐ Fortakehl ® (Penicillium roquefortii) – tabs 4X - **1 tab twice weekly**.

☐ Mucokehl ® (Mucor racemosus) – tabs 5X - **1 tab twice weekly**.

☐ Nigersan ® (Aspergillus niger) – tabs 5X - **1 tab twice weekly**.

☐ Notakehl ® (Penicillium chrysogenum) – tabs 5X - **1 tab twice weekly.**

☐ Pefrakehl ® (Candida parapsilosis) – Caps 4X - **1 cap twice weekly**.

If there is vaginal discharge, or anal Candida, then vaginal or anal pessaries of Albicansan D3 must also be used to eliminate this topical infection. These can be used every second day last thing at night, after sex and are shown on the table above with the symbol　☐ .

The SANUM remedies are continued for 10 weeks until the end of the Candida protocol.

These remedies are taken BEFORE or AWAY from food, this is why it is best to store them in the bedroom, away from electrical equipment, and take them as soon as you wake in the morning, and last thing at night.

There are both capsules and tablets. The capsules you need to open and pour the powder that they contain under the tongue and allow it to absorb for a few minutes. The tablets dissolve under the tongue for a few minutes – no water needs to be drunk, as they will absorb directly into the blood stream from the blood vessels under the tongue.

1. **ALBICANSAN** - European health practitioners report that this remedy may be useful as supportive therapy in:

☐ intestinal overgrowth of Candida

☐ mycosis

☐ resistant skin infections of mouth

☐ stomatitis

☐ gingivitis

☐ urogenital mycosis

☐ vaginitis

☐ urethritis with subsequent adnexitis

☐ cholecystitis

☐ colitis of fungal origin

☐ allergies

2. **FORTAKEHL** - European practitioners report that Fortakehl apparently promotes normal bowel flora in the gastro-intestinal tract (especially after antibiotic therapy) which could be helpful for such conditions as gastritis, enteritis, colitis, gall bladder problems, pancreatitis, diarrhea, constipation, ulcers, yeast infections of the intestines, the vagina, and the skin.

3. **MUCOKEHL** - European health practitioners report that this remedy is useful as supportive therapy in chronic and acute disturbances of circulatory system, such as:

☐ thrombosis

☐ embolism

☐ angina pectoris

☐ post infarct

☐ varicosities

☐ hemorrhoids

☐ diabetic gangrene and neuropathy

☐ constipation.

4.**NIGERSAN** - European health practitioners report that this remedy is useful in disorders that have to do with disturbed calcium metabolism which could involve bone and tooth rehabilitation. European reports further indicate that Nigersan, also known as Pleo™ Nig has been successfully used for urogenital tract problems in men and women such as prostate, ovaries, kidney and bladder complaints. It appears to be helpful for enhancing lymph circulation which in turn leads to increased detoxification, especially after illness.

5. **NOTAKEHL** - European practitioners report that Notakehl, otherwise known as Pleo™ Not is very useful to enhance the immune system, and as a supportive therapy for infections of bacterial origin and inflammations such staph, strep, acne, ear infections, tonsil infections, sore throat, neuritis, neuralgia, urinary tract infections, prostate irritation, respiratory infections and neuropathy.

6. **PEFRAKEHL** - European health practitioners report that Pefrakehl, otherwise known as Pleo™ Pef may be useful as a supportive therapy in relieving the symptoms of intestinal overgrowth of Candida, yeast infections, mycosis, fungal, bacterial and viral infections of the mouth and the teeth, ear infections, gingivitis, urogenital yeast infections, vaginal yeast infections, anal inflammations and irritations.

N.B. Please note that if you are allergic to PENICILLIN, you should not take the NOTAKEHL (Penicillium chrysogenum) and FORTAKEHL (Penicillium roquefortii) as these are likely to cause unpleasant symptoms such as lethargy, fatigue, brain fog, muscle pains and a general feeling of unwellness. The treatment will still work without these two SANUM remedies.

Phase 5 - Balancing Body Chemistry

It is a commonly recognized and accepted fact that immune system efficiency is highly dependent on the proper biochemical balance in the body. This of course, is dependent on proper and adequate nutrition to supply the body with all the required biochemical constituents (vitamins, minerals, enzymes, intrinsic factors, etc.).

Different people require different amounts and balances of nutrients for optimum health. The criteria for the determination of these differing nutritional requirements lies within the definition of one's metabolic type, i.e., the genetically determined metabolic and nutritional parameters that define each person's individuality on every level.

It is precisely because different people have different metabolic types, and therefore different needs for nutrition, that the allopathic, symptom-treatment approach in nutrition is baseless and so often ineffective. This further explains why what (nutritionally) helps make one person better, may have little or no effect on another, or even make a third person worse.

I have not tried to modify this protocol as I have found it to be so successful in the treatment of over 5,000 patients to date, that I dare not juggle with it in case it loses its effectiveness. I'm sure that it can be improved upon and would welcome comments from other practitioners working with Candida. It is only through sharing that we will grow and become better practitioners [23,24].

---

[23] Georgiou, G.J. Scourge of the 21st Century: Systemic Candidiasis – Part 1. British Naturopathic Journal, Vol. 25, No. 1, 2008.
[24] Georgiou, G.J. Treatment of Systemic Candidaisis – Part 2. British Naturopathic Journal, Vol. 25, No. 1, 2008.

Package of All Supplements Required for the Da Vinci Candida Protocol

If you purchase the DA VINCI CANDIDA PROTOCOL – COMPLETE PACKAGE of supplements from www.worldwidehealthcenter.net you will receive the following products to last you throughout the complete treatment over 3 months.

☐ 6 containers of CANDA PLUS

☐ 3 containers of HOROPITO + ANISEED

☐ 3 containers of CAPRYLATE

☐ 3 containers of ACIDOPHILUS AND BIFIDUS

☐ 1 container of CANDIDA 30 C

☐ SANUM REMEDIES – complete set for 3 months (6 packs in total) containing Nigersan D5, Pefrekehl D4, 1 x Albicansan D4, Fortakehl D5, Notakehl D5, Mucokehl D5.

☐ All handouts required giving detailed instructions, written and used by Dr. Georgiou at the Da Vinci Center. Handouts include: "Da Vinci Candida Protocol"; "Sanum Remedies"; "Anti-Candida Diet"; "Candida Meal Plan". These can be downloaded as soon as you purchase the package.

Reintroducing Fruit

Fruit can be re-introduced back into the diet FOUR WEEKS after you begin taking the SANUM remedies, or 6 weeks after beginning the Candida protocol.

Stay with two SOLID portions of fruit daily for the remainder of the protocol. One medium apple would be considered as one portion – or

½ teacup of berries would be one portion, or 2 small plums would be one portion.

All JUICY fruits such as watermelon, grapes, oranges, grapefruit, tangerines, mangos, pineapple and very sweet figs should be avoided throughout the 3 months of the treatment as they give their sugars to the blood too quickly. Stick with apples, pears, plums, ½ cup of berries, kiwi, paw-paw – have these in between meals as snacks, one mid-morning and one mid-afternoon.

Herxheimer Reactions

Depending on the severity of Candida overgrowth and the amount of the agents taken, the Candida can be killed off in vast numbers in a very short period of time. As the fungi are killed, they release substances that are toxic to the body – these are called mycotoxins. If the elimination organs such as the kidneys, liver, lymphatics, gut and skin cannot clear these mycotoxins quickly and they accumulate in the tissues, then a temporary toxic or allergic-type reaction can occur. The technical name for this experience is a 'Herxheimer reaction'; it is more commonly referred to as "die off."

Usually die-off lasts about 12 – 24 hours, though on rare occasions it can last several days. It can usually be controlled by reducing the dosage of the remedies used to kill the Candida, as well as taking drainage herbs and homeopathics that your practitioner will advise you of.

Signs of Herxheimer reaction can be many and varied but generally involve such discomfort as aching, bloating, dizziness, nausea, and an overall "goopy sick" feeling, or a worsening of original symptoms. Fortunately, die off is generally short in duration, and although uncomfortable, is at least a confirmation of the presence of Candida and that something "good" is happening.

Exercise as well as ensuring proper, daily bowel evacuation has been reported as being helpful in countering the adversities of die off. Maintaining a high daily intake of pure water is also important to keep the channels of elimination open. Sometimes taking a teaspoon of baking soda (sodium bicarbonate) in a glass of water can help to quickly neutralize acidic reactions in the body that lead to inflammation and pain.

It may be possible to slow down these symptoms, many of which are caused by acetaldehyde, one of the main toxins produced by yeast. Taking Molybdenum – 10 drops x 2 times daily in water, away from food can break down this toxin into something far less harmless. It may be worth considering adding these to the Candida protocol if Herxheimer reactions are bad.

The Blocking Factors of Recovery – Reasons for Failing

Depending on the severity of Candida overgrowth and the amount of the agents taken, the Candida can be killed off in vast numbers in a very short period of time. As the fungi are killed, they release substances that are toxic to the body – these are called mycotoxins. If the elimination organs such as the kidneys, liver, lymphatics, gut and skin cannot clear these mycotoxins quickly and they accumulate in the tissues, then a temporary toxic or allergic-type reaction can occur. The technical name for this experience is a 'Herxheimer reaction'; it is more commonly referred to as "die off."

Usually die-off lasts about 12 – 24 hours, though on rare occasions it can last several days. It can usually be controlled by reducing the dosage of the remedies used to kill the Candida, as well as taking drainage herbs and homeopathics that your practitioner will advise you of.

Signs of Herxheimer reaction can be many and varied but generally involve such discomfort as aching, bloating, dizziness, nausea, and an overall "goopy sick" feeling, or a worsening of original symptoms. Fortunately, die off is generally short in duration, and although uncomfortable, is at least a confirmation of the presence of Candida and that something "good" is happening.

Exercise as well as ensuring proper, daily bowel evacuation has been reported as being helpful in countering the adversities of die off. Maintaining a high daily intake of pure water is also important to keep the channels of elimination open. Sometimes taking a teaspoon of baking soda (sodium bicarbonate) in a glass of water can help to quickly neutralize acidic reactions in the body that lead to inflammation and pain.

It may be possible to slow down these symptoms, many of which are caused by acetaldehyde, one of the main toxins produced by yeast. Taking Molybdenum – 10 drops x 2 times daily in water, away from food can break down this toxin into something far less harmless. It may be worth considering adding these to the Candida protocol if Herxheimer reactions are bad.

Natural Antibiotics During the Candida Protocol

It is critical that anyone on the 3-month Candida protocol stock-up on NATURAL ANTIMICROBIAL PACK that they might require if they come down with a cold, flu, sore throat or any kind of infection while they are still on the Candida protocol.

These natural antibiotics have been tried and tested for many years and seem to work fine with most infections. However, it is very important to take these immediately when the first symptoms appear. If you leave the infection for a couple of days, the microbes will spread quickly and it will be more difficult to shift it with the natural antibiotics.

This is why it is critical to have these natural antibiotics in your medical dispensary BEFORE beginning the Candida protocol. They have an expiry date of between two and five years, so you will no doubt use them during this time.

The dosages mentioned below are for adults. For maximum effectiveness it is good to use at least four of the natural antibiotics mentioned below, all in combination together.

These natural antibiotics and herbal supplements include the following that have been used successfully in clinical practice, and in fact have been used by all my family for over 30 years, given that none of my 4 children have ever taken antibiotics in their life!

1.GRAPEFRUIT SEED EXTRACT (**Citricidal™**): Is a very effective anti-fungal, available in tablet form as well as liquid form which can be placed under nails with fungus. Take 2 tablets 3 times daily. For nails, one drop under each nail morning and evening.

2.OREGANO OIL: If one is citrus intolerant, then you can use Oregano oil gel capsules instead – 1 gel capsule 3 times daily.

3.SILVER LIQUID 50 ppm (colloidal silver) – You can take 1 – 3 teaspoons, 3 times daily.

4.VITAMIN C – Take either 2 caps (1000 mg each) 3 times daily, or ½ teaspoon 3 times daily of the calcium ascorbate powder form.

5.PARAFORM PLUS TWO – this contains a broad spectrum of active herbals, probiotics and other natural cleansing and protective agents, which have anti-bacterial, anti-fungal, anti-microbial and anti-inflammatory actions. Take one cap x 3 times daily.

There is no reason why ALL these should not be combined together, but in the least, 4 of the 5 should be combined for maximum effectiveness. Please do not underestimate the importance and value of stocking up on these natural antimicrobials. We have prepared a

NATURAL ANTIMICROBIAL PACK in our one-stop shop for your convenience (www.worldwidehealthcenter.net).

I have seen on a few occasions, patients that I was treating for Candida not stocking these natural antibiotics and they came down with a nasty bug that went deep into the lungs within days. By the time they could obtain all these remedies, their symptoms had reached a level where they had to see a medical practitioner, who rightly so, prescribed antibiotic drugs.

It is touch and go whether the Candida protocol will succeed or not when taking antibiotic drugs. The problem is that the antibiotics will inevitably kill off the good bacteria in the gut as well as the bad, and if this creates a severe enough dysbiosis, then the pathogenic, hyphal forms of Candida will begin to proliferate again.

This is very sad when you must announce to the patient that they have to extend their Candida protocol for another month or longer – very frustrating!

CHAPTER 7:

My Own Case Studies from Patients Cured

There is still a lot of controversy around the topic of Candida, and I am the first to agree that we do not have all the answers. One thing that I have witnessed in clinical practice, however, is the astounding recovery that many of these so-called Candidiasis patients make when placed on the Da Vinci Candida Protocol (DCP).

Personally, I have seen many different skin problems clear when the systemic Candidiasis is treated including psoriasis, as well as chronic sinusitis, joint pains, cheloids or scar formations, splitting skin on hands, chronic coughs and sore throats of many years standing, chronic thrush and vaginal discharge, headaches and migraines, chronic fatigue or myalgic encephalomyelitis (ME) and many other rather atypical symptoms that were labeled as "Idiopathic" which basically means "unknown etiology." Here are a few case histories for your interest:

Case 1

This is a case of a woman who went in for a D & C scrape of the uterus and the gynecologist ruptured the uterus and she required emergency surgery due to heavy internal hemorrhage. She received a number of IV antibiotics and a couple of months after being discharged she suffered from splitting hands along with chronic thrush, fatigue and other skin rashes of unknown origin. She made a dramatic improvement in all these symptoms after completing the Da Vinci Candida Protocol.

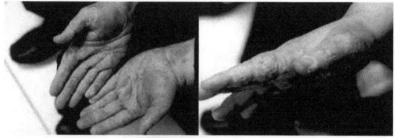

Case 1: Bad case of splitting hands after IV antibiotics

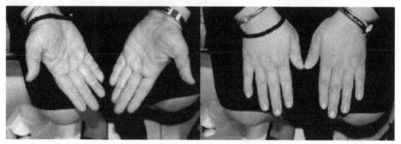

Case 1: Two-months into the Da Vinci Candida Treatment

Case 2

This is a lady that had suffered from chronic psoriasis for over 20 years – this had spread to most of her torso as well as limbs. One of the underlying problems of the skin problem was systemic Candidiasis which cleared after three months of the Da Vinci Candida Protocol.

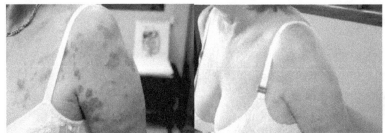

Case 2: Chronic psoriasis (left) and 3-months after completion of Da Vinci Candida Treatment

Case 3

A complex case of an idiopathic skin problem of 20 years' duration. Using the Candida Treatment Protocol resulted in over 75% improvement, but there was a bacterial element that needed further treatment to eliminate it.

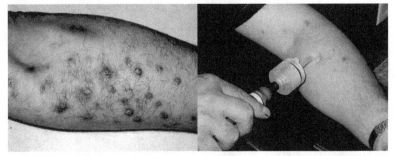

Case 3: Idiopathic skin problems of 20-years duration (left) and after treatment (right)

Case 4

A young adult who had contracted herpes and Steven-Johnson Syndrome during blood infusions – when presented for treatment he was in excruciating pain, had lost 8 kg and was tube feeding. Treatment using the Candida Treatment Protocol eliminated this difficult problem.

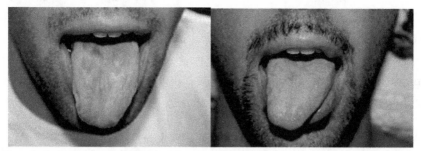

Case 4: Complex case with underlying Candida (left) and one month into treatment (right)

Other Clinical Cases

Here are a few more cases that I have seen in clinical practice – each has different symptoms, yet one of the major underlying factors was Systemic Candidiasis.

Case No. 1: Mrs. A, Age 44

Mrs. A's presenting symptoms were somewhat unusual in that she continually complained that she frequently had the sense of a strong fishy odor in her nostrils over the last 7 years.

She remembers that this began when she had cleaned mold in her house with chlorine – the mold had appeared after a flood.

She also suffered from many allergies which included allergy to flowers, bananas and melon.

Her main symptoms apart from the annoying fishy odor was, constant intermittent coughing as well as a heavy pressure-type sensation in the chest and lungs. She had clear signs of nail fungus as well as frequent vaginal discharge.

She had consulted a number of medical doctors and dermatologists, but with no success. The dermatologist gave her antifungal cream for the nails. The condition remained as before.

She underwent Bioresonance diagnosis using the VEGA system and was found to have a number of food intolerances too such as: wheat, lactose and milk products, bananas, caffeine, sugar, chicken, pork, nightshade family of vegetables (potatoes, tomatoes, peppers, and aubergines), olive oil and olives.

The VEGA test also showed that she was resonating with pathological, mycelial forms of Candida albicans, indicating that she was suffering from systemic Candidiasis – mixed molds were also found during this testing protocol.

It was decided to help her body to detox and return back to an alkaline pH, as well as help eliminate inflammatory chemicals and other toxins. She followed an alkaline detoxification diet for 2 weeks based on alkaline foods such as fruit and vegetables.

Her energy levels after the detox had tremendously increased and she reported clarity of mind. She began the Da Vinci Candida Protocol for 3 months – see main text for details.

The smell of fish had decreased by 30% in intensity and the frequency to cough had also decreased by 40% within the first 3 weeks of the protocol treatment. After two months of treatment, the cough had improved 60%.

Previously she would cough for one hour, now she coughs less than one minute. The smell of fish has improved by 70%.

After the completion of the Candida protocol (3 months), the Candida finally disappeared, and the cough had improved by 100%. This was the first time that the cough had improved in the past 7 years. The smell of fish had also vanished as well as the nail fungus on her toes – this was also helped by adding grapefruit seed extract liquid – one drop per nail morning and evening. She was a very happy woman!

Case No. 2: Mr. M, Age 45

Mr. M presented with a chronic cough that he had for the past 7-8 years, accompanied by whitish phlegm. He was diagnosed with H. Pylori for which the medical doctor prescribed antibiotics which were taken on and off for a period of 2 years. The coughing however persisted even though he had consulted many doctors, including ENT (otolaryngologists) and pneumologists with no results.

Before coughing began, he lived in a moldy apartment.

He underwent VEGA food intolerance testing that showed intolerance to a number of foods such as: wheat, soya, lactose and milk products, beans, caffeine, almonds and walnuts, pork, citrus (lemon, grapefruit, and oranges), olive oil and olives. He is a vegetarian but includes lactose and fish in his diet.

The VEGA testing also showed that he was suffering from systemic Candida albicans. He followed an alkaline detoxification diet for 15 days based on fruit and vegetables. During the detox the cough had decreased by 50% in frequency and 70% decrease in intensity. The white phlegm had stopped completely.

Immediately after the detox he began the Da Vinci Candida protocol for 3 months. During the Candida protocol his energy levels had massively increased, and he had incredible clarity of mind.

After the Candida treatment, his cough had completely vanished, and the phlegm decreased to minimum.

Case No. 3: Mrs. S, Age 49

Mrs. S complained that she had bronchial asthma and suffered from allergies. Medical doctors gave her cortisone sprays. She also suffered from obesity (147 kg) and whenever she tried to diet, she suffered from hypoglycemia.

Other health issues included atrial fibrillation (cardiac arrhythmia) and GERD- gastroesophageal reflux disease. She was taking Warfarin, an anticoagulant, to prevent blood clots from forming. She was also taking medication to control her arrhythmia.

She had also removed her thyroid nodules and was taking thyroxine daily.

It was recommended that she begin with a compromised alkaline detoxification diet lasting 1 month. This means that the body will be detoxing slower than the 15 days alkaline detox diet by leaving in protein foods the first two weeks. This procedure is recommended when there are chronic degenerative diseases, in order to prevent any possible adverse reactions caused by the elimination of inflammatory chemicals.

So, the first week of detox she was allowed to eat fish and pulses along with fruit and vegetables. The second week the fish was eliminated and only the pulses remained along with the fruit and vegetables. During the final two weeks she only ate fruit and vegetables.

During the detox her stomach digestion improved, and she was feeling much better; edema had also disappeared after some heavy urination initially, and she had lost noticeable inches around her waist – to her delight as weight loss had been blocked for a long time.

During Bioresonance testing it was shown that she was intolerant to a number of foods such as: wheat, lactose and milk products, citrus (oranges, lemons, grapefruits), caffeine, sugar, hazelnut, walnuts, almonds, pork, chicken, and nightshade family of vegetables (potatoes, tomatoes, aubergines, peppers).

In addition, the Vega Bio-dermal testing also showed that she was suffering from systemic Candidiasis. She therefore began the Da Vinci Candida protocol for 3 months. During the Candida protocol, she had lost a total of 12 kg, her asthmatic symptoms had gone completely, and she could now climb steps without wheezing and panting, being much quicker on her feet. As an added gift, her chronic sinusitis had also completely cleared.

CONCLUSIONS

This brings us to the end of the book on how to *genuinely and safely* cure your Candida. In my clinical experience over the last 35 years, I have witnessed people turning around their health using the Da Vinci Candida Protocol – it truly gives me a lot of Spiritual satisfaction to see people that have suffered for many years get better <u>in only 3 months</u>.

Therefore I decided to write this book, in order to share with everyone a successful way to treat your Candida. I certainly would not have written the book if I did not have a rich experience in treating Candida with many *thousands* of patients throughout the years.

There is a difference talking theoretically about treatments, and being on the front lines with many patients and witnessing how they recover from so many ailments.

So, I dedicate this book to my many patients that have patiently worked with me and taught me so many things included in this book – I bless you all with good health and happiness!

APPENDIX

Dr. Crooks Candida Questionnaire

If you would like to know if your health problems are yeast-related, take this comprehensive test. Questions in Section A focus on your medical history-factors that promote the growth of Candida albicans and that are frequently found people with yeast-related health problems. In Section B, you will find a list of 23 symptoms that are often present in patients with yeast-related health problems. Section C consists of 33 other symptoms that are sometimes seen in people with yeast-related problems – yet they may also be found in people with other disorders.

Filling out and scoring the questionnaire should help you and your physician evaluate the possible role that candida albicans plays in your health problems.

SECTION A: HISTORY

•Have you ever taken tetracycline, or other antibiotics, for acne for one month or longer? (points 35)

•Have you, at any time in your life, taken broad-spectrum antibiotics or other antibacterial medication for respiratory, urinary or other infections for two months or longer, or in shorter courses four or more times in a one-year period?   (Points 35).

•Have you taken a broad-spectrum antibiotic drug even in a single dose?   (points 6)

•Have you at any time in your life been bothered by persistent prostatitis, vaginitis or other problems affecting your reproductive organs? (points 25)

•Are you bothered by memory or concentration problems do you sometimes feel spaced out? (points 20)

•Do you feel "sick all over", yet despite visits to many different physicians the cause has not been found? (points 20)

•Have you been pregnant two or more times? (points 5)

• One time? (points 3)

• Have you taken birth control pills for more than two years? (points 15)

• For six months to two years? (points 8)

• Have you taken steroids orally, by injection or inhalation for more than two weeks? (points 15)

• For two weeks or less? (points 6)

•Does exposure to perfume, insecticides, fabric shop odors and other chemicals provoke symptoms? Moderate to severe (points 20) Mild (points 5)

• Does tobacco smoke really bother you? (points 10)

• Are your symptoms worse on damp, muggy days or in moldy places? (points 20)

• Have you had athlete's foot, ring worm, jock itch or other chronic fun-gal infections of the skin or nails? Severe or persistent (points 20) Mild to moderate (points 10)

• Do you have crave sugar? (points 10)

TOTAL SCORE SECTION A _____

SECTION B: MAJOR SYMPTOMS

For each of your symptoms, enter the appropriate figure in the pint score column.

1. If a symptom is occasional or mild   **3 points**

2. If a symptom is frequent and/ or moderately severe   **6 points**

3. If a symptom is severe and/ or disabling   **9 points**

Add total score and record it at the end of this section.

• Fatigue or lethargy   _____

• Feeling of being "drained"   _____

• Depression or manic depression   _____

• Numbness, burning or tingling   _____

• Headache   _____

• Muscle aches   _____

• Muscle weakness or paralysis   _____

• Paint and/ or swelling in joints   _____

• Abdominal pain   _____

• Constipation and/ or diarrhoea   _____

• Bloating, belching or intestinal gas   _____

• Troublesome vaginal burning, itching or discharge   _____

- Prostatitis   _____

- Impotence   _____

- Loss of sexual desire or feeling   _____

- Endometriosis or infertility   _____

- Cramps and/ or other menstrual irregularities   _____

- Premenstrual tension   _____

- Attacks of anxiety or crying   _____

- Cold hands or feet, low body temperature   _____

- Hypothyroid   _____

- Shaking or irritable when hungry   _____

- Cystitis or interstitial cystitis   _____

TOTAL SCORE, SECTION B   _____

SECTION C: OTHER SYMPTOMS

For each of your symptoms, enter the appropriate figure in the point score column.

1.If a symptom is occasional or m   **3 points**

2.If a symptom is frequent and/ or moderately severe   **6 points**

3.If a symptom is severe and/ or disabling   **9 points**

Add total score and record it at the end of his section.

- Drowsiness, including inappropriate drowsiness   _____

- Irritability   _____

- In coordination   _____

- Frequent mood swings   _____

- Insomnia   _____

- Dizziness/ loss of balance   _____

- Pressure above ears, tenderness of cheekbones or

forehead   _____

- Tendency to bruise easily   _____

- Eczema, itching eyes   _____

- Psoriasis   _____

- Chronic hives (urticaria)   _____

- Indigestion or heartburn   _____

- Sensitivity to milk, wheat, corn or other common foods   _____

- Mucus in stools   _____

- Rectal itching   _____

- Dry mouth or throat   _____

- Mouth rashes, including "white" tongue   _____

- Bad breath   _____

- Foot, hair or body odour not relieved by washing   _____

- Nasal congestion or postnasal drip   _____

- Nasal itching   _____

• Sore throat   _____

• Laryngitis, loss of voice   _____

• Cough or recurrent bronchitis   _____

• Pain or tightness in chest   _____

• Wheezing or shortness of breath   _____

• Urinary frequency or urgency   _____

• Burning on urination   _____

• Spots in front of eyes or erratic vision   _____

• Burning or tearing eyes   _____

• Recurrent infections or fluid in ears   _____

• Ear pain or deafness   _____

TOTAL SCORE, SECTION C   _____

GRAND TOTAL (SECTION A, B AND C)   _____

The **Grand Total Score** will help you and your physician decide if your health problems are yeast-connected. Scores in women will run higher, as seven items in the questionnaire apply to women, while only two apply exclusively to men.

• Yeast –connected health problems are almost certainly present in women with scores of **more than 180**, and in men with of **more than 140.**

•Yeast-connected health problems are probably present in women with scores of **more than 120**, and in men with scores **more than 90.**

•Yeast-connected health problems are possibly present in women with scores of **more than 60**, and in me of **more than 40.**

• With scores of less than 60 in women and 40 in men, yeasts are less apt to be the cause of health problems.

Score of 60-99 yeast a possible cause of health problems
Score of 100-139 yeast a probable cause of health problems.
Score of 140 or more yeast almost certainly a cause of health problems

PARASITE QUESTIONNAIRE

These are many causes for each symptom listed below. Assign points to each symptom and see if a pattern develops.

A= Symptom never occur
B= Symptom occurs occasionally
C= Symptom occurs frequently
D= Symptom occurs regularly

Questions	A	B	C	D
Restless sleep	0	1	2	3
Skin problems, rashes, itches	0	1	2	3
Increased appetite, hungry after meals	0	1	2	3
Frequent diarrhea, loose stools	0	1	2	3
Grinding of teeth when asleep	0	1	2	3
Variable, changeable consistency of stools	0	1	2	3
Picking of nose, boring nose with finger	0	1	2	3
Abdominal pains	0	1	2	3
Vertical wrinkles around mouth	0	1	2	3
Rectal, anal itching	0	1	2	3
Parallel lines (tracks) in soles of feet	0	1	2	3
Intestinal cramps, burning	0	1	2	3

Irritability (no apparent reason)	0	1	2	3
Feeling bloated, gaseous	0	1	2	3
Diarrhea alternating with constipation	0	1	2	3
Bowel urgency, occasional accidents	0	1	2	3
Hyperactive tendency (nervous)	0	1	2	3
Dark circles under eyes	0	1	2	3
Need for extra sleep, waking unrefreshed	0	1	2	3
Allergies, food sensitivities	0	1	2	3
Fevers of unknown origin	0	1	2	3
Night sweats (not menopausal)	0	1	2	3
Kissing pets, allowing them to lick your face	0	1	2	3
Anaemia	0	1	2	3
Frequent colds, flu, sore throats	0	1	2	3
Going barefoot in parks, public streets	0	1	2	3
Travelling in 3rd countries	0	1	2	3
Eating lightly cooked pork products	0	1	2	3
Eating sushi, sashimi	0	1	2	3
Sleeping with pets on bed	0	1	2	3
Bed wetting	0	1	2	3
Men: sexual dysfunction	0	1	2	3
Forgetfulness	0	1	2	3
Slow reflexes	0	1	2	3

	Loss of appetite	0	1	2	3
	Yellowish face	0	1	2	3
	Heart beat rapid	0	1	2	3
	Heart pain	0	1	2	3
	Pain in the umbilicus	0	1	2	3
	Blurry, unclear face	0	1	2	3
	Pain: back, thighs, shoulders	0	1	2	3
	Lethargy, apathy	0	1	2	3
	Numbness, tingling in hands, feet	0	1	2	3
	Burning pains in the stomach, intestines	0	1	2	3
	Menstrual problems	0	1	2	3
	Dry lips during day, damp at night	0	1	2	3
	Drooling while asleep	0	1	2	3
	Occult blood in stool (shown from lab tests)	0	1	2	3
	History of giardia, pin worms, other worms	0	1	2	3
	Swimming in creeks, rivers, lakes	0	1	2	3

Total score

10-14 points = maybe parasite infestation

15- 20 points = suspect parasites

22-25 points = likely- (Further testing helpful)

25 or more = parasites involvement high likely

REFERENCES

Al-Doory Y. 1969. The mycology of the freeliving baboon (Papio sp.). Mycopathologia et Mycologia Applicata 38: 7–15.

Anderson KE, Kappas A. Dietary regulation of cytochrome P-450. Annu Rev Nutr. 11:141-167, 1991.

Ballie-Hamilton, P. The Detox diet. UK: Penguin, 2002.

Banerjee, M., D.S. Thompson, A. Lazzell, P.L. Carlisle, C. Pierce, C. Monteagudo, J.L. Lopez-Ribot, and D. Kadosh. 2008. UME6, a novel filament-specific regulator of Candida albicans hyphal extension and virulence. Mol. Biol. Cell 19, 1354-1365.

Barclay GR, McKenzie H, Pennington J, Parratt D, Pennington CR. The effect of dietary yeast on the activity of stable chronic Crohn's disease. Scand J Gastroenterol 1992; 27 :196–200.

Bartlett JG, Gilbert DN, Spellberg B. Seven ways to preserve the miracle of antibiotics. Clin Infect Dis. 2013;56(10):1445–1450.

Bastidas RJ, Heitman J: Trimorphic stepping stones pave the way to fungal virulence. PNAS 2009; 106: 351–2.

Berman J: Morphogenesis and cell cycle progression in Candida albicans. Curr Opin Microbiol 2006; 9: 595–601.

Bernhardt H, Knoke M. Mycological aspects of gastrointestinal microflora. Scand J Gastroenterol 1997; 32(suppl 222) :102–106.

Bland JS, Bralley JA. Nutritoinal upregulation of hepatic detoxification enzymes. J Appl Nutr. 44(3&4):2-15, 1992.

Blankenship, J.R. and A.P. Mitchell. 2006. How to build a biofilm: a fungal perspective. Curr. Opin. Microbiol. 9, 588-594.

Brandtzaeg P. The mucosal B cell and its functions. In: Brostoff J, Challacombe S (eds): Food Allergy and Intolerance. London: Saunders; 2002:127-171.

Budtz- Jorgensen, E. Cellular immunity in acquired Candidiasis of the palate. Scand. J. Dent. Res. 81, 372, 1973

Cabot, S. Juice Fasting Detoxification. USA: The Sprout House, 1992.

Calderone RA, Fonzi WA: Virulence factors of Candida albicans. Trends Microbiol 2001; 9: 327–35.

Calderone, R.A., and R.L. Cihlar (e.d.). Fungal pathogenesis: principles and clinical applications. Marcel Dekker, Inc., New York, N.Y, 2002

Carlisle, P.L., M. Banerjee, A. Lazzell, C. Monteagudo, J.L. LopezRibot, and D. Kadosh. 2009. Expression levels of a filament-specific transcriptional regulator are sufficient to determine Candida albicans morphology and virulence. Proc. Natl. Acad. Sci. USA 106, 599-604.

Centers for Disease Control and Prevention, Office of Infectious Disease Antibiotic resistance threats in the United States, 2013. Apr, 2013. Available at: http://www.cdc.gov/drugresistance/threat-report-2013. Accessed January 28, 2015.

Crampin, H., K. Finley, M. Gerami-Nejad, H. Court, C. Gale, J. Berman, and P.E. Sudbery. 2005. Candida albicans hyphae have a Spitzenkorper that is distinct from the polarisome found in yeast and pseudohyphae. J. Cell. Sci. 118, 2935-2947.

Crandall M. The pathogenetic significance of Intestinal Candida Colonization, 2004

Crook WG: The yeast connection, A medical Breakthrough 2nd Addition Professional Books, Jackson, TN, 1984

Crook, WG. The Yeast Connection and the Woman. Professional Books, Jackson TN 1987.

Dalkilic E, Aksebzeci T, Kocatürk I, Aydin N, Koculu B: The investigation of pathogenity and virulence of Candida. In: Tümbay E, Seeliger HPR, Ang

Ö (eds.): Candida and Candidamycosis. New York: Plenum Press 1991; 50: 167–74

Davies MH, Gough A, Sorhi RS, Hassel A, Warning R, Emery P. Sulphoxidation and sulphation capacity in patients with primary biliary cirrhosis. J Hepatol. 22(5):551-560, May 1995.

Douglas LJ: Candida biofilms and their role in infection. Trends Microbiol 2003; 11: 30–6.

Enderlein, G. (1925). Bakterien-Cyclogenie, Verlag de Gruyter & Co, Berlin.

Filler SG, Sheppard DC: Fungal invasion of normally non- phagocytic host cells. PLOS Pathog. 2006; 2: e129.

Fitzsimmons N, Berry DR. Inhibition of Candida albicans by Lactobacillus acidophilus : evidence for the involvement of a peroxidase system. Microbios 1994; 80 :125–133.

Gail Burton. Candida - The Silent Epidemic, Candida Causative factors, 4-9, 2003

Georgiou, G.J. (2008) British Naturopathic Journal, Vol. 25.,No. 1 & 2.

Georgiou, G.J. (2005) Explore! Volume 14, No. 6.

Grant DM. Detoxification pathways of the liver. J Inher Metab Dis. 14;421-430, 1991.

Grubb SEW, Murdoch C, Sudbery PE, Saville SP, Lopez-Ribot JL, Thornhill MH: Candida albicans-endothelial cell interactions: a key step in the pathogenesis of systemic candidiasis. Infect Immun 2008; 76: 4370–7.

Hesseltine HC, Campbell LK. 1938. Diabetic or mycotic vulvovaginitis. American Journal of Obstetrics and Gynecology 35: 272–283.

Hornby, J.M., E.C. Jensen, A.D. Lisec, J.J. Tasto, B. Jahnke, R. Shoemaker, P. Dussault, and K.W. Nickerson. 2001. Quorum sensing in the dimorphic fungus Candida albicans is mediated by farnesol. Appl. Environ. Microbiol. 67, 2982-2992

Hube B: From commensal to pathogen: stage- and tissue-specific gene expression of Candida albicans. Curr Opin Microbiol 2004; 7: 336–41.

Hulda Regehr Clark, Ph.D., N.D., The Cure for all Diseases 1995

Hussein, H.S., and J.M. Brasel. Toxicity, metabolism, and impact of mycotoxins on humans and animals. Toxicology 167, 2001

Iwata, K.; Yamamoto, Y "Glycoprotein Toxins Produced by Candida albicans." Proceedings of the Fourth International Conference on the Mycoses, PAHO Scientific Publication #356, June 1977.

John Parks Trowbridge, M.D., and Morton Walker, D.P.M., The yeast syndrome- Antibiotics Encourage Yeast Overgrowth, 45-46, 1986

Kanda N, Tani K, Enomoto U, Nakai K & Watanabe S. The skin fungus-induced Th1- and Th2-related cytokine, chemokine and prostaglandin E 2 production in peripheral blood mononuclear cells from patients with atopic dermatitis and psoriasis vulgaris. Clinical & Experimental Allergy; 32(8):1243-50.

Kennedy MJ, Volz PA. Ecology of Candida albicans gut colonisation: inhibition of Candida adhesion, colonisation and dissemination from the gastrointestnal tracy by bacterial antagonism. Infect Immun 1985; 49: 654–63.

Koivikko A, et al.. Allergenic cross-reactivity of yeasts. Allergy 1988; 43:192-200.

Kubo I, Fujita K, Lee SH, Ha TJ. Antibacterial activity of polygodial. Phytother Res. 2005 Dec;19(12):1013-7.

Kumamoto CA, Vinces MD: Alternative Candida albicans lifestyles: growth on surfaces. Annu Rev Microbiol 2005; 59: 113–33.

Lee SH, Lee JR, Lunde CS, Kubo I. In vitro antifungal susceptibilities of Candida albicans and other fungal pathogens to polygodial, a sesquiterpene dialdehyde. Planta Med. 1999 Apr;65(3):204-8.

Leon Chaitow N.D, D.O, Candida Albicans- Could yeast be your problem? How Candida gets out of hand. Chapter 3- Immune System Deficiency, 24-26, 1991

Lushniak BD. Antibiotic resistance: a public health crisis. Public Health Rep. 2014;129(4):314–316.

Luyt CE, Brechot N, Trouillet JL, Chastre J. Antibiotic stewardship in the intensive care unit. Crit Care. 2014;18(5):480.

Magee PT, Chibana H: The genomes of Candida albicans and other Candida species. In: Calderone RA (ed.): Candida and candi - diasis. Washington: ASM Press 2002; 293–304

Michael T. Murray, N.D., Chronic Candidiasis, Dietary factors, sugar and the yeast syndrome: 43,44, 1997

Morschhäuser J, Köhler G, Ziebuhr W, Blum-Oehler G, Dobrindt U, Hacker J: Evolution of microbial pathogens. Phil Trans R Soc Lond 2000; 355: 695–704.

Morita E, Hide M, Yoneya Y, Kannbe M, Tanaka A, Yamamoto S: An assessment of the role of Candida albicans antigen in atopic dermatitis. J Dermatol 1999; 26: 282–7. 20. Pappas PG, Rex JH, Sobel JD, et al.: Guidelines for treatment of Candidiasis. CID 2004; 38: 161–89. 21.

Netea MG, Brown GD, Kullberg BJ, Gow NAR: An integrated model of the recognition of Candida albicans by the innate immune system. Nat Rev Immunol 2008; 6: 67–78.

Nieuwenhuizen WF, Pieters RH, Knippels LM, Jansen MC, Koppelman GJ. Is Candida albicans a trigger for the onset of coeliac disease? Lancet 2003; 361 :2152–2154.

Nobile, C.J. and A.P. Mitchell. 2006. Genetics and genomics of Candida albicans biofilm formation. Cell. Microbiol. 8, 1382-1391

Noverr MC, Falkowski NR, McDonald RA, McKenzie AN , Huffnagle GB: Development of allergic airway disease in mice following antibiotic therapy and fungal microbiota increase: role of host genetics, antigen, and interleukin-13. Infect Immun 2005; 73: 30–8.

Noverr MC, Phare SM, Toews GB, Coffey MJ, Huffnagle GB: Path - ogenic yeasts Cryptococcus neoformans and Candida albicans produce immunomodulatory prostaglandins. Infect Immun 2001; 69: 2957–63.

Noverr MC, Noggle RM, Toews GB, Huffnagle GB: Role of antibiotics and fungal microbiota in driving pulmonary allergic responses. Infect Immun 2004; 72: 4996–5003.

Odds FC. 1988. Candida and Candidosis, 2nd edn. Bailli`ere Tindall: London.

Piddock LJ. The crisis of no new antibiotics—what is the way forward? Lancet Infect Dis. 2012;12(3):249–253.

Piispanen AE, Hogan DA: PEPped up: induction of Candida albicans virulence by bacterial cell wall fragments. Cell Host Microbe 2008; 4: 1–2

Polakova S, Blume C, Zarate JA, Mentel M, Jorck-Ramberg D, Stenderup J, et al.: Formation of new chromosomes as a virulence mechanism in yeast Candida glabrata. PNAS 2009; 106: 2688–93

Poulain D, Hopwood V, Vernes A. Antigenic variability of candida albicans. CRC Crit Rev Microbiol 1985; 12:223-70.

Raska M, Belakova J, Krupka M, Weigl E: Candidiasis – Do we need to fight or to tolerate the Candida fungus? Folia Microbiol 2007; 52: 297–312.

Reinel D, Plettenberg A, Seebacher C, et al.: Orale Candidose. Leitlinie der Deutschen Dermatologischen Gesellschaft und der Deutschsprachigen Mykologischen Gesellschaft. JDDG 2008; 7: 593–7.

Reinholdt J, Krogh P, Holmstrup P. Degradation of IgA1, IgA2, and S-IgA by candida and torulopsis species. Acta Path Microbiol Immunol Scand, Sect C 1987; 95:65-74.

Romani L, Bistoni F, Puccetti P. Initiation of T-helper cell immunity to Candida albicans by IL-12: the role of neutrophils. Chem Immunol. 1997; 68:110-35.

Romani L, Bistoni F, Puccetti P: Adaptation of Candida albicans to the host environment: the role of morphogenesis in virulence and survival in mammalian hosts. Curr Opin Microbiol 2003; 6: 338–43.

145

Salloum, TK. Fasting Signs and Symptoms: A Clinical Guide. USA: Buckeye Naturopathic Press, 1992.

Scrivner, J. Detox Yourself. UK: Judy Piatkus (Publishers) Ltd., 1998.

Seelig MS. Mechanisms by which antibiotics increase the incidence and severity of candidiasis and alter the immunological defences. Bacteriol Rev 1 1966; 30 :4442–4459.

Shah DT, Jackman S, Engle J, Larsen B. Effect of gliotoxin on human polymorphonuclear neutrophils. Inf Dis Obster Gynecol 1998; 6 :168–175.

Shen J, Cowen LE, Griffin AM, Chan L, Kohler JR: The Candida albicans pescadillo homolog is required for normal hypha-to-yeast morphogenesis and yeast proliferation. PNAS 2008; 105: 20918–23.

Soll DR: Phenotypic switching. In: Calderone RA (ed.): Candida and Candidiasis. Washington: ASM Press 2002; 123–42.

Sudbery, P.E., N.A.R. Gow, and J. Berman. 2004. The distinct morphogenic states of Candida albicans. Trends Microbiol. 12, 317- 324

The Chronic Candidiasis Syndrome: Intestinal Candida and its relation to chronic illness OAM 1996-1997, 16. Gutierrez, J.; Maroto, C. et al: Circulating Candida antigens and antibodies: useful markers of candidemia. Journal of Clinical Microbiology. 31(9):25502, 1993.

Thewes S, Kretschmar M, Park H, Schaller M, Filler SG, Hube B: In vivo and ex vivo comparative transcriptional profiling of invasive and noninvasive Candida albicans isolates identifies genes associated with tissue invasion. Mol Microbiol 2007; 63: 1606–28.

Trowbridge JP and Walker M. The yeast Syndrome Bantam Books, New York, N.Y, 1986

Truss C: The missing Diagnosis Birmingham Alabama (The Author), 1983

Truss, CO. Metabolic abnormalities in patients with chronic Candidiasis - the acetaldehyde hypothesis, Journal of Orthomolecular Medicine, 13:63- 93, 1984

Viswanathan VK. Off-label abuse of antibiotics by bacteria. Gut Microbes. 2014;5(1):3–4.

Vojdani A, Rahimian P, Kalhor H and Mordechai E. Immunological cross reactivity between candida albicans and human tissue. J Clin Lab Immunol 1996; 48:1-15.

Wade, C. Inner Cleansing: How to Free Yourself from the Joint-Muscle-Artery-Circulation Sludge. New York: Parker Publishing Co., 1992.

Walsh, TJ.; Lee, JW.; et al: "Serum Darabinitol measured by automated quantitative enzymatic assay for detection and therapeutic monitoring of experimental disseminated candidiasis: correlation with tissue concentrations of Candida albicans." Journal of Medical & Veterinary Mycology. 32(3):20515, 1994.

Weig M, Werner E, Frosh M, Kasper H. Limited effect of refined carbohydrate dietary supplementation on colonization of the gastrointestinal tract of healthy subjects by Candida albicans . Am J Clin Nutr 1999; 69 :1170–1173.

William G. Crook, M.D., Chronic Fatigue Syndrome and the yeast connection, Probiotics: 260,261, 1992

William G. Crook, M.D., The yeast connection - Candida questionnaire and score sheet - Diagnosis of a yeast-Related disorder, 29-33, Food allergies: 122, 1986

Xu XL, Lee RTH, Fang HM, Wang YM, Li R, Zou H, et al.: Bacterial pepti doglycan triggers Candida albicans hyphal growth by directly activating the adenylyl cyclase cyr1p. Cell Host Microbe 2008; 4: 28–39

Videos

If you wish to watch some webinars and videos that I have done about Candida and others, here they are (if you cannot see the link, just search on YouTube for "Dr. Georgiou and Candida":

Candida Videos:

https://www.youtube.com/watch?v=nOYIFKrGbrM&t=620s

https://www.youtube.com/watch?v=VQnE8VQXEpc

Disclaimer

The information contained within this book is offered for you to make educated health decisions so that you can optimize your health. If there are serious health conditions, then you should always consult your primary care physician before beginning any other treatment regime.

The health information in this book is not advice and should not be treated as such – it is provided without any representations or warranties, express or implied. We do not warrant or represent that the medical information in this book is true, accurate, complete, current or non-misleading.

You must not rely on the information in this book as an alternative to medical advice from your doctor or other professional healthcare provider. If you have any specific questions about any medical matter, you should consult your doctor or other professional healthcare provider. If you think you may be suffering from any medical condition, you should seek immediate medical attention. You should never delay seeking medical advice, disregard medical advice or discontinue medical treatment because of information in this book.

While every attempt has been made to provide information that is both accurate and cutting-edge, the author cannot be held responsible for any decision that the reader may take while reading the guide, nor can a guarantee be provided that this guide and the remedies that it recommends will help everyone.

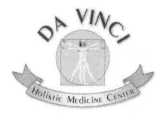

Tel: +357 24 – 82 33 22
Email:
admin@naturaltherapycenter.com
Web: www.naturaltherapycenter.com

Clinical Consultations

To book appointments to see Dr Georgiou at the Da Vinci Holistic Health Center in Larnaca, Cyprus simply call the Center or email.

Da Vinci Institute of Holistic Medicine

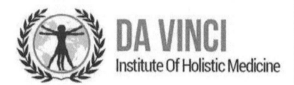

Tel: +357 24 – 82 33 22
Email:
admin@collegenaturalmedicine.com
Web: www.collegenaturalmedicine.com

Holistic Medicine Education

Anyone interested in completing studies in Holistic Medicine can apply directly to the Da Vinci Institute of Holistic Medicine.

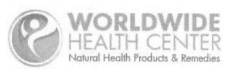

Tel: +357 24 82 33 22
Email: admin@worldwidehealthcenter.net
Web: www.worldwidehealthcenter.net

Natural Supplements

Most of the supplements mentioned in this book can be obtained from this website.

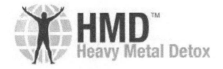

Tel: + 357 24 82 33 22
Email: admin@detoxmetals.com
Web: www.detoxmetals.com

Heavy Metal Detox

Products related to the natural detox of toxic metals can be purchased here - sent globally.

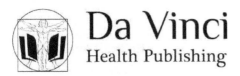

Tel: + 357 24 82 33 22
Email: admin@davincipublishers.com

Ethical Publishing

Health practitioners that want to publish their books, but do not want to lose their copyright, while gaining most of the royalties, can apply to Da Vinci Health Publishing – the ethical publishers!

ABOUT THE AUTHOR

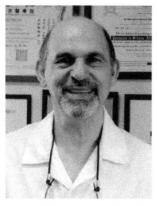

Dr. George John Georgiou, 62 years old, has 11 degrees and Diplomas spanning 25 years in various topics ranging from Biology, Psychology and Natural Medicine. Specifically:

1. Bachelor of Science (B.Sc) honours degree in Biology/Psychology from Oxford Brook's University, Oxford, England
2. Master's of Science degree (M.Sc) in Clinical Psychology from the University of Surrey, Guildford, England
3. Doctor of Philosophy degree (Ph.D). in Clinical Sexology from The Institute for Advanced Study of Human Sexuality, San Francisco, USA.
4. Doctor of Science (D.Sc (AM)) degree in Alternative Medicine from the International Open University of Alternative Medicine
5. Clinical Nutrition (Dip.ION - Distinction) from the Institute of Optimum Nutrition (ION), London, England
6. Diploma in Electronic Impulse Therapy (Dip.E.I.Th) from the Euro College of Complementary Medicine, UK
7. Diploma in Naturopathic Iridology from the Holistic Health College, UK and Diploma in Iridology from the Society of Iridologists, UK
8. Diploma as a Master Herbalist (MH) from the Holistic Health College, UK
9. Diploma in Homeopathic Medicine (DIHom) from the British Institute of Homeopathy, UK
10. Diploma in Su Jok Acupuncture from Onnuri College, Almaty, Kazakhstan
11. Doctor of Naturopathic Medicine (Pastoral) – N.D. (P) from the Sacred Medical Order of the Knights of Hope, US – Licence number: L1016988.

He is the Director Founder of the Da Vinci Holistic Health Centre in Larnaca, Cyprus – see www.naturaltherapycenter.com   This is a multimodality centre specializing in treating chronic diseases of all kinds. This model of healthcare using a holistic approach has been illustrated in his 23 books that he has written to date.

Research is also one of his passions and he is considered an expert in natural heavy metals detoxification, having been awarded a Doctor of Science in this topic. He has spent over three years formulating and testing using double-blind, placebo-controlled trials with over 350 people a natural toxic metal chelator called HMD™ (Heavy Metal Detox). He is presently the worldwide patent-pending holder on this product which is sold worldwide at www.detoxmetals.com

There are many papers that Dr Georgiou has published in peer-reviewed journals that are available on his websites at www.naturaltherapycenter.com and www.detoxmetals.com

Dr Georgiou has also been Knighted as a Knight Hospitaller by the Sovereign Medical Order of the Knights Hospitaller (www.smokh.org), one of the oldest Christian charitable organizations in the world with over 200 medical knights all practicing holistic medicine using natural medicine formulated by the monks of old practicing monastic medicine. They have built 5 hospitals and clinics worldwide all running on charitable donations to help the poor. As the Diplomatic Cultural Attache for Cyprus he is presently in the process of setting up the St. Luke's Health Care Charity to help people in need through Holistic Medicine.

His research interests have made him the Principle Investigator for the World Health Organization (WHO) in studies on AIDS and Drug Use, as well as other research involving alcoholism, drug abuse and sexual dysfunctions. He has lectured to Master's students in Psychology at an external campus for Indiana University, USA, and has been a prolific writer of health articles for the general public, having written literally thousands in both English and Greek languages.

Regarding his career in Clinical Sexology, he was the first professional sexologist to ever work in Cyprus, making history in this respect. This was back in 1983 when sexology was unheard of in this sexually repressed country.

His doctoral dissertation in Clinical Sexology was entitled *The Sexual Attitudes of Greek Orthodox Priests* – a unique study never before studied in the Orthodox religion. There was considerable antagonism from certain spheres of the Orthodox Greek church regarding the results of the study.

In 1990 he had his own live radio programme on Saturday lunchtime entitled *Human Sexuality.* This was far ahead of its time and in a two-year period Dr Georgiou managed to cover 96 topics of human sexuality with the audience asking questions reflecting the ignorance, taboos and prejudices of the time. This was the first such programme in the history of Cyprus.

In 1999 he published the first book ever written in the Greek language on the treatment of Premature Ejaculation, published in Greece. He is also the Editor for the chapter on Cyprus in the International Encyclopedia of Sexuality, Volume 4.

As Dr Georgiou has two doctorates, one in Clinical Sexology and one in Alternative Medicine, he has formulated protocols for the treatment of sexual dysfunctions that involve the integration of both these disciplines. He has coined this *Naturopathic Sexology* which is a unique term pertinent to himself – if you Google this term it will bring you back to his websites.

He is presently the Director Founder of the Da Vinci Holistic Health Center[2] in Larnaca, Cyprus, as well as the Academic Director of the Da Vinci Institute of Holistic Medicine,[3] a distance-learning educational institution, and the Director/founder of the Da Vinci BioSciences Research Center.

---

[2] www.naturaltherapycenter.com
[3] www.collegenaturalmedicine.com

He is a Member of the following Associations/Institutes:

- The Society of Biology, UK (MSBiol.)
- Chartered Biologist, UK (C. Biol)
- Member of the Royal Microscopy Society, UK
- The General Council and Register of Naturopaths, UK (GCRN)
- Full Member, The British Naturopathic Association, UK
- Member of Oncology Group, British Naturopathic Association
- The Register of Naturopathic Iridologists, UK (M.R.N.I.)
- The British Association of Nutritional Therapists, UK (BANT)
- The Association of Master Herbalists, UK. (AMH)
- Fellow of the British Institute of Homeopathy, UK (FBIH)
- The American College of Clinical Thermology, USA
- The International Su Jok Therapy Association, Russia
- The British Holistic Medical Association, UK (BHMA)
- Member of the Institute of Complementary Medicine, UK (ICM)
- National Iridology Research Association, USA (NIRA)
- Associate Fellow of the British Psychological Society, UK (AFBPsS)
- Chartered Psychologist, UK, BPS (C.Psychol)
- Member, Health Professions Council, UK – registered as Clinical Psychologist (PYL15128)
- Member of Cyprus Psychologists' Association, Cyprus.
- Diplomate of the American Board of Sexology, USA (ABS)
- Registered Sex Therapist with ABS, USA
- Member, The American College of Sexologists, USA (ACS)
- Fellow of the American Academy of Clinical Sexologists, USA (FAACS)
- Member, World Association for Sexology (WAS), USA
- Member of the Cyprus Association of Alternative Therapists (N.D.).

Dr. Georgiou is married to Maria, a Psychotherapist/Lecturer and has 4 children aged between 18 and 31 years, and grandchildren. His hobbies and interests include flying a private plane, classic antique motorbike and car restoration, antique furniture restoration, horology, playing the bouzouki, web master, travelling, writing, researching, bee keeping and running an organic farm.

More Books written by Dr Georgiou:

1. Surviving a Nuclear War: Save Your Family and Loved Ones
2. Gallstones: Ridding Stones Naturally in 24 Hours
3. Diabetes: Natural Treatments that Really Work – Latest Research!
4. Crohn's Disease: Heal Naturally Without Medication
5. Reflux Disease: Natural Healing for GERD in 90 Days
6. Lupus: Let Nature Heal – Find Out How
7. Haemorrhoids: The Natural Cure
8. Cholesterol: Heal Naturally Without Medication – Many Secrets Revealed!
9. Diverticulosis: Natural Healing That Works
10. Why Am I Sick? Eliminate the Causes and Be Well Forever!

CPSIA information can be obtained
at www.ICGtesting.com
Printed in the USA
LVHW050445230520
656338LV00006B/614